W9-BZO-021

Sick to Death

and Not Going to Take It Anymore!

CALIFORNIA/MILBANK BOOKS ON HEALTH AND THE PUBLIC

Sick to Death

and Not Going to Take It Anymore!

REFORMING HEALTH CARE FOR THE LAST YEARS OF LIFE

Joanne Lynn

University of California Press
BERKELEY   LOS ANGELES   LONDON

Milbank Memorial Fund
NEW YORK

The Milbank Memorial Fund is an endowed operating foundation that engages in nonpartisan analysis, study, research, and communication on significant issues in health policy. In the Fund's own publications, in reports or books it publishes with other organizations, and in articles it commissions for publication by other organizations, the Fund endeavors to maintain the highest standards for accuracy and fairness. Statements by individual authors, however, do not necessarily reflect opinions or factual determinations of the Fund.

University of California Press
Berkeley and Los Angeles, California

University of California Press, Ltd.
London, England

© 2004 by the Regents of the University of California

Library of Congress Cataloging-in-Publication Data

Lynn, Joanne, 1951–
   Sick to death and not going to take it anymore! : reforming health care for the last years of life / Joanne Lynn.
       p.   cm. — (California/Milbank books on health and the public ; 10)
   Includes bibliographical references and index.
   ISBN 0-520-24300-5 (alk. paper).
       1. Older people—Medical care—United States.   2. Older people—Long term care—United States.   3. Chronically ill— Medical care —United States.   4. Terminal care—United States.   5. Health care reform—United States. [DNLM: 1. Chronic Disease—Aged—United States.   2. Terminal Care—Aged—United States.   3. Health Care Reform—United States.   4. Health Services for the Aged—United States.   5. Long-Term Care—Aged—United States.   WT 500 L989s 2004]   I. Title.   II. Series.
   RA564.8.L973   2004
   362.198'97'00973—dc22   2004010910

Manufactured in the United States of America

13   12   11   10   09   08   07   06   05   04
10   9   8   7   6   5   4   3   2   1

Printed on Ecobook 50 containing a minimum 50% post-consumer waste, processed chlorine free. The balance contains virgin pulp, including 25% Forest Stewardship Council Certified for no old growth tree cutting, processed either TCF or ECF. The sheet is acid-free and meets the minimum requirements of ANSI/NISO Z39.48–1992 (R 1997) *(Permanence of Paper)*.

Contents

Illustrations and Tables

Figures

Tables

Foreword

The Milbank Memorial Fund is an endowed operating foundation that engages in nonpartisan analysis, study, research, and communication on significant issues in health policy. Since 1905 the Fund has worked to improve and maintain health by encouraging persons who make and implement health policy to use the best available evidence. The Fund convenes meetings of leaders in the public and private sectors and publishes reports, articles, and books.

This is the tenth of the California/Milbank Books on Health and the Public. The publishing partnership between the Fund and the University of California Press seeks to encourage the synthesis and communication of findings from research that could contribute to more effective health policy.

Joanne Lynn is a pioneering clinician in geriatric medicine, an innovative researcher, and an inspiring speaker. Throughout her distinguished career, she has emphasized that the care received by people who are approaching the end of life requires considerable improvement and reorganization from the moment they are diagnosed as having a serious chronic disease.

In recent years, Lynn and her colleagues have conducted extensive research on the experience of persons with severe chronic disease. They also have supported scores of clinical teams trying to improve the services they offer. This research and its pragmatic applications led Lynn to organize data and services around a small number of trajectories of the course of major groups of diseases. These trajectories are models confirmed by the analysis of substantial data. Lynn also assessed the care that patients currently receive as they live these trajectories. This assessment revealed remarkable shortcomings in the usual approaches to care for people nearing the end of life. The most obvious of these flaws are inadequate treatment of pain and other symptoms, ineffectual prevention of disabilities and lack of support for people who must live with disabilities, and insufficient guidance to patients and their families in organizing financial and living arrangements.

This book builds on Lynn's research and that of others to describe how, in her words, "health care and community services simply do not meet the needs of the large number of people facing a prolonged period of progressive illness and disability before death." Because American society does not "even have the language with which to discuss" this phase of life, physicians and other health professionals and the media too often ignore it.

In this book, Lynn combines knowledge based on research with passionate advocacy of an agenda for far-reaching reforms. She is precise about how policy makers and health professionals could improve care for the growing number of persons with severe chronic disease—and how reliable care could be in place in time for the aging of the baby boom.

Daniel M. Fox
President

Samuel L. Milbank
Chairman

Acknowledgments

This book grew from the work of Americans for Better Care of the Dying and the draft of a report commissioned by the Milbank Memorial Fund in 2000. That manuscript received extensive reviews from a variety of concerned experts, and their critiques have greatly shaped its transition to a book. The strong guiding hand of the president of the Milbank Memorial Fund, Dan Fox, has been central to envisioning and completing the work. I am grateful also for the financial support of the Milbank Memorial Fund and the Washington Home Center for Palliative Care Studies.

I am especially indebted to those who reviewed the manuscript in its draft as a report: Julia Addington-Hall, Gerard Anderson, Robert Arnold, Amos Bailey, Barry Baines, Patricia Barry, Robert Berenson, Richard Brumley, Kenneth Brummel-Smith, Melinda Beeuwkes Buntin, Helen Burstin, Robert Burt, Ira Byock, Margaret Campbell, Ronald Carson, Christine Cassel, Jean Chabut, Myra Christopher, Stephen Connor, LaVera Crawley, June Dahl, Marion Danis, Karen Davie, Richard Della Penna, Sandra DiPasquale, Bruce Doblin, Bob Doherty, Ken Doka, Garey Eakes, Thomas Edes, Paul Elstein, Linda Emanuel, Susan Emmer, David English, Gilbert Fanciullo, Betty Ferrell, Perry Fine, Joseph Fins, Thomas Finucane, Kathleen Foley, Nicole Makosky Fowler, Nancy Freeborne, Linda Fried, Terri Fried, Jon Gabel, Barbara Gage, Rosemary Gibson, Muriel Gillick, Paul Glare, Shimon Glick, Susan Goldwater, Jack Gordon, David Gould, Michelle Grant-Ervin, James Hallenbeck, Mary Beth Hamel, Joan Harrold, Elma Holder, Scott Hopes, Ed Howard, Thomas Hoyer, Lisa Iezzoni, David Introcaso, Amber Jones, Stan Jones, Judith Kitzes, Mary Jane Koren, Harlan Krumholz, Howard Lerner, Thomas A. Louis, James Lubitz, Janice Lynch, Cheryl Cox Macpherson, Patricia MacTaggart, Marianne Laporte Matzo, Kathy McMahon, Diane Meier, Robin Meili, Tracy Miller,

Velvet Miller, Mary Mologne, Marilyn Moon, Charles Mouton, Don Murphy, Isobel Murray, Linda Norlander, Jean Oberstar, Joseph O'Neill, Marilyn Pattison, L. Gregory Pawlson, Kate Payne, Timothy Quill, Raymond Rawson, Donna Regenstreif, Michael Rodgers, Susan Rogers, Kenneth Rosenfeld, Peggy Rosenzweig, Judy Ryan, Charles Sabatino, Steven Schroeder, J. Donald Schumacher, Charles Scott, Lisa Shugarman, Andrew Smith, Mildred Solomon, Emese Somogyi-Zalud, Claire Tehan, William Thar, Ed Thomas, Jim Towey, Wayne Ury, Charles von Gunten, Neil Wenger, Terrie Wetle, Josh Wiener, and Shin-Yi Wu.

I am also especially indebted to those who reviewed the manuscript in its expanded version as a book: Christine Cassel, Kathleen Foley, Lisa Iezzoni, Diane Meier, and Marilyn Moon.

I would further like to thank Robert Brook, Vicki Freedman, Mary Lerner, Ann O'Mara, Charles Palmer, Peggy Parks, Russell Phillips, Donna Regenstreif, Corinne Rieder, and Bobby Silverstein for their helpful guidance on specific aspects or sections.

My book builds upon the insights of many who are working hard to build the care system of the future. All who aim to improve care for those living with fatal chronic illness are especially indebted to the Open Society Institute, which sponsored the Project on Death in America, and the Robert Wood Johnson Foundation, which sponsored a series of projects in end-of-life care and chronic conditions from 1988 through 2003.

I have the great good fortune to work with three extraordinary organizations, where colleagues have been loyal supporters of the research that has gone into this book. I am especially indebted to Robert Brook and Sarah Myers at RAND Health; Cria Gregory, Maureen Lilly, Sharon Love, Hsien Seow, and Anne Wilkinson at the Washington Home Center for Palliative Care Studies; and Roshon Gibson and Janice Lynch Schuster at Americans for Better Care of the Dying.

INTRODUCTION

The life stories of most Americans nowadays are long and remarkably free from serious disability or disease. When serious disability, progressive chronic illness, or frailty arrives, it is usually only in the last chapters of our life stories. Growing old before becoming seriously ill and dying is a remarkable accomplishment. Just a century ago, serious illnesses and disabilities were common at every age, and dying was usually quick.

Yet long life poses its own challenges. Health care and community services simply do not meet the needs of the large number of people facing a prolonged period of progressive illness and disability before death. American society doesn't even have the language with which to discuss this previously uncommon phase of life. The subject gets little coverage in the news media and little attention in popular culture, leaving us without shared stories to make sense of our situation. Dysfunctions that result from outdated health-care and social arrangements cause fear and suffering for most of us, both when we try to help a family member or friend with a fatal illness and when we ourselves are ill. Sometimes a person dies peaceably and gracefully at the end of a long life. Everyone concerned considers this person to have been "lucky"—precisely because all of us know that the last part of life so often includes untreated pain, financial disaster, loss of control, frustrating struggles with disabilities, and even a generally miserable and purposeless last chapter.

It doesn't have to be this way. Most people can live well with serious, eventually fatal chronic illnesses, whether for a few months or for many years. When supportive services ensure that very sick and disabled people coming to the end of life can count on being comfortable and comforted, we ordinarily have highly meaningful experiences in the time that is left.

Why can't we all have a good ending? Why can't we count on good care when we need it most? Why do we tolerate a health-care system that leaves people in pain, confused, bankrupted, demeaned, and frightened? We could do much better—and we should. The reforms that we need are within our grasp. What we need most is a shared vision of good care, innovative approaches for achieving this vision, and the will to make the changes happen.

For twenty-five years now, I have struggled to find care arrangements that would let ordinary Americans live through their last years with comfort, dignity, and human meaningfulness. This quest has taken various forms: I have served a few thousand dying people as their personal physician; shared in the work of dedicated and skilled teams caring for seriously ill persons at home and in nursing homes; encouraged the spread of hospice services to every corner of the nation; written legal briefs to courts that were confronting difficult cases; participated in substantial research projects; led quality improvement in scores of care-provider organizations; and written guidance books for patients and families. These multiple roles have taught me much about the complexity of the current health-care system and the urgency of change. They also have let me learn from a variety of skilled and thoughtful colleagues who share the goals of service to those living with serious illness. Many of my insights here reflect the growing base of knowledge already garnered and the creative initiatives already undertaken. These efforts have had substantial effect; but I am now convinced that we need to reform public policy and reshape social arrangements in order to enjoy reliably good care in the last years of life.

This book aims to provide the essentials for those reforms—facts, perspectives, goals, and strategies. This is an owner's manual for the health-care system, for all of us who expect to live long and die well. As citizens, we own the health-care system that we will have to use when we are sick and dying, especially since it mostly relies on public funds. When "care" is profoundly unreliable, as it is now, we have the right and the obligation to fix it. A dedicated effort will teach us the rest of what we need to know, and successful reforms could quickly make this book as outdated as our care system is now. All of us face the prospect of serious chronic illness in our last years, and all of us have a stake in engineering reform. What will it take?

First, we need a better understanding of what the future holds and what can be done—we need to "face the facts." We can't count on our changes being improvements without having a solid grasp of the situation that confronts us.

Second, we need to think creatively, interpret information in new ways, and imagine untried possibilities.

Third, we need to learn what arrangements actually work well, both from existing "gems" and from deliberate trials of innovations.

Fourth, we need to identify the opportunities and challenges that our history, culture, and social arrangements provide—some suitable to build upon and others to leave behind.

Finally, we must implement high-leverage reforms aimed at broad improvement, both reengineering the services and marshaling the political mandate to overcome complacency.

That is the outline of this book: facts, concepts, examples, strategies, and implementation. What I cannot supply is the energy and commitment to make change happen, because that requires you, putting your efforts into this cause. We can do it. We can have a reliable care system that lets us live meaningfully and comfortably despite serious illness in our last years. Nothing is in the way, except habit and inattention. Surely, as we anticipate the harsh experience of caring for a loved one in a dysfunctional system, or of scraping through the last part of our own lives with inept services, we can overcome the inertia of accepting current arrangements. We all have to live out our days using the care system that we establish. We will deserve the suffering we get, if we leave the situation unchanged.

I

JUST THE FACTS

Serious Chronic Disease in the
Last Phase of Life

Just a few generations ago, serious illness, like hazardous weather, arrived with little warning, and people either recovered or worsened and died within days or weeks. People had a great deal of trouble from illnesses that are now nearly eradicated—such things as childbirth complications, improperly healed fractures, broken teeth, and parasites. Nevertheless, the calamity that caused death was rarely apparent even a week or two ahead of death. Had they not encountered the specific illness or injury that overtook them, most of those who died could have lived for many years. A working man would die of his first heart attack or a young mother of childbirth fever. Our images of health and disease and our health-care system arose in that setting—where people reasonably thought that death had a single cause and that preventing it was the obvious yardstick of successful health care. The usual life story has changed a great deal, but our outdated health-care system is not equipped to handle its new challenges.

Health care for individuals, along with public health, now prevents or cures many of the illnesses and injuries that abbreviated the lives of our ancestors, effectively allowing most Americans to live into old age. Indeed, most of the burden of illness and use of health-care services now fall in the last phase of life, when people generally deal with established, serious, eventually fatal chronic illnesses for a few years. In their younger years, people have two dominant priorities for health care: prevention and cure of illness. But as people come to the end of a long life today, prevention of serious illness is no longer possible, and neither is cure. Instead, that part of life generates very different priorities, including symptom prevention and relief, support of family members, plans for future care, enhancement of dignity, and completion of life projects.

Most Americans today have long lives; more than 75 percent live past age sixty-five (Hogan et al. 2000). In fact, 83 percent of Americans now die while covered by Medicare (people who are older than sixty-five and also younger people with certain long-term disabilities or renal failure) (Hogan et al. 2000). During the last century, the life span of Americans nearly doubled. In 2000, the average life expectancy was eighty years for American women and seventy-four years for American men, compared to an average of just forty-nine years in 1900 (National Center for Health Statistics 2002, 33). By 2050, life expectancy for women and men will likely increase to eighty-four and eighty, respectively (Institute for the Future 2000).

Back in 1900, only a very few people lingered for years with a disability arising from eventually fatal chronic illness. Most died from infections and accidents, and the time from onset of serious disability to death was measured in hours or weeks, not years. Two serious chronic illnesses caused most long-term, life-shortening disability: tuberculosis and mental illness. Many persons with either condition were segregated into sanatoriums and no longer participated in the life of the wider community. In contrast, Americans today can expect to spend a few years living with serious disability at the end of life, and disability and death will again become a part of everyday life. From the start of the twentieth century to its final decade, the top ten causes of death shifted remarkably, as illustrated in table 1.

Improved public health interventions and medical treatments have meant that very few now die from childbirth, workplace accidents, epidemic infections, or their first heart attack. Instead, Americans live with serious progressive disease for years, and 70 percent of us die from chronic cardiovascular disease, cancers, diabetes, or strokes (Centers for Disease Control and Prevention 1999).

Table 1. *Top ten causes of death, 1900 and 2000*

Rank	1900	2000
1	Pneumonia	Heart disease
2	Tuberculosis	Cancer
3	Diarrhea and enteritis	Stroke
4	Heart disease	Emphysema and chronic bronchitis
5	Liver disease	Unintentional injuries
6	Injuries	Diabetes
7	Stroke	Pneumonia and influenza
8	Cancer	Alzheimer's disease
9	Senility	Kidney failure
10	Diphtheria	Septicemia

Sources: For 1900, U.S. Department of Health and Human Services 2000, 22. For 2000, National Center for Health Statistics 2001.

In addition to changes in life span and duration of illness before death, caregiving and treatment too have changed, as reflected in the following comparison (National Center for Health Statistics 2002):

	1900	2000
Age at death	Forty-seven years	Seventy-five years
Usual place of death	Home	Hospital
Coverage for most medical expenses	Family	Medicare
Disability before death	Usually not much	Two years, on average

Compared to a century ago, not only are people today less likely to die from acute causes early in life, but they are also less likely to get all their care from family members and more likely to require care outside the home. Some of these changes originated in the broader social commitment to Medicare and the potential for more treatments in the hospital. In addition, long-term disability has generated greater needs than many families can handle on their own. Especially as the age of serious illness and death has come later, the spouses and children who provide care have also become older and often are disabled themselves.

Living with Chronic Conditions

A medical school professor, aiming to orient my class to the medical profession thirty years ago, claimed, "Office practice is mainly cuts, sore throats, and the worried well." He may have been overstating the case even then, but he certainly would be wrong now. Most of medical care has become the care of chronic conditions. Nearly half of all Americans have one or more chronic conditions, which generally require some accommodations in order to get through the day and some ongoing upkeep to prevent or delay worsening or disability (Anderson, Horvath, and Anderson 2002). Currently, about forty million people, or 15 percent of the adult U.S. population, are limited in activities as a result of a chronic health condition (Kaye et al. 1996). Of these, almost 5 percent have difficulty walking (Freedman and Martin 1998); 7–8 percent have severe cognitive impairments (Freedman, Aykan, and Martin 2001); and 20 percent have impaired vision (Desai et al. 2001). With advancing age, the likelihood of disability gets much higher (Fried and Guralnik 1997). After age eighty-five, only one person in twenty is still fully mobile (Sharma et al. 2001). Age and disability are the strongest factors in predicting further declines in functioning, recurrent hospitalization, institutionalization, and death, even after taking into account other personal characteristics such as smoking, obesity, and several specific chronic diseases (Corti et al. 1994; Manton, Corder, and Stallard 1993).

Of those living with any chronic condition, most are suffering from more than one (Wolff, Starfield, and Anderson 2002). In the Medicare population, the average beneficiary sees seven different physicians and fills upwards of twenty prescriptions per year (Anderson, Horvath, and

Anderson 2002). Having multiple chronic conditions puts people at greater risk of disability, activity limitations, and high costs. The health-care cost for a person older than sixty-five averages three to five times greater than the cost for an average younger person.

Even so, for Medicare populations with various levels of serious chronic conditions at age seventy, the costs of medical care for the rest of life are remarkably similar (Lubitz et al. 2003). A seventy-year-old healthy person with no functional limitations will spend about $136,000 in Medicare-covered services (hospitals, physicians, rehabilitation, durable equipment) during a life expectancy of fourteen more years, living with a functional limitation for six of those additional years. A seventy-year-old who is limited in at least one activity of daily living (such as mobility, toileting, feeding) will spend an average of about $145,000 in Medicare coverage during a life expectancy of twelve more years, having a functional limitation for nearly eight years of that time. Most Americans do not yet recognize the impact of these figures: even the healthy person at age seventy is in for many years of living with a disability, and length of life does not make much difference in the costs per person in Medicare. Yet since the use of institutional long-term care increases steeply with advancing age, the costs that Medicare does not cover will increase sharply with longer survival.

Most elderly people have accumulated some combination of arthritis, hearing or vision problems, dental decay or malfunction, painful feet, sluggish bowels, and urinary difficulties. Most people live for many years with such conditions, which worsen only gradually. Chronic conditions like these incur substantial costs, as well as symptoms and functional challenges; but they don't generally cause serious dependency or death.

An important group of chronic conditions, in contrast, regularly worsen and eventually cause death. Overwhelmingly, these are cancer, organ system failure (heart, lung, liver, or kidney, mostly), dementia, and stroke. Nine out of ten elderly who die covered by Medicare have one or more of these conditions in the year preceding death (Hogan et al. 2000). Most of us eventually get one or more of these conditions; however, at any one time, only a small proportion of people have these serious conditions, probably about one-quarter to one-third of the elderly (Lynn and Adamson 2003). Thus, both of these statements are true: most elderly are healthy, *and* virtually all Americans will have a substantial period of serious illness and disability before death.

Cognitive disability and frailty are rapidly becoming dominant elements of dying in old age, even though they are hard to track because these conditions are not reliably identified and recorded. Already, half of Americans who die past age eighty-five (and one-third of us live that long) have major memory loss as part of their final phase of life (Cornoni-Huntley et al. 1985). The proportion is lower at younger ages, though still commonplace. This cognitive loss can arise from Alzheimer's dementia, strokes, Parkinson's disease, and other syndromes. The course early on usually allows the person to be active, but lapses in judgment, memory, and self-control require constant supervision. Later on, the person often becomes unable to move about, use the toilet, or otherwise provide for self-care. From that time to the end of life, someone else must assist with every bodily function. The course usually lasts for years. Since cognitive loss is strongly correlated with age, as more of the population lives to old age, more will have cognitive deficits as part of the challenges posed.

Frailty is, in effect, the fragility of multiple body systems as their customary reserves diminish with age and disease. Instability when walking, problems with vision and hearing, loss of muscle strength, and lack of reserve in critical organ systems (heart and lung, especially) are typical elements (Fried et al. 2001; Gillick 2001). While people with substantial frailty may stay mentally capable, they still need help with daily activities and are at constant risk of major calamities like hip fractures, pneumonia, falls, strokes, and infections. Partly from outliving peers but also from incurring deficits in hearing and mobility, frail persons often become socially isolated and unhappy, especially if they have to leave familiar surroundings to move into nursing homes. Their spouses are often as old and frail, or already deceased, and their children are themselves getting old, so no family helper may be available or sufficient. Frailty is probably already a major pathway through the last part of life, but the standard classifications of illness do not provide for it and hence often misleadingly count persons with this general state of decline as having "heart failure" or some other specific manifestation.

Indeed, our coding and classifications are generally misleading for those with serious chronic conditions at the last phase of life. Most Americans have a number of years of good health in old age, but usually the accumulation of chronic conditions gradually causes progressive disabilities and limits the person's ability to overcome setbacks. Younger people have substantial reserves and can often overcome major illnesses, but old and frail people with chronic illnesses exist in a very fragile balance with the demands of their environment and often cannot withstand even small threats to that balance. Living with serious illness or frailty in old age is like walking on a high wire, and the cause of the final stumble and fall is mischaracterized when it is termed the "cause of death," since being out on the high wire itself is what makes the stumble lethal. Less metaphorically, being in a fragile state of health for a long time at the end of life is what makes colds, flu, pneumonia, falls, and other modest setbacks into common causes of death. We misunderstand the situation when we count the incidental cause as being lethal, when it is really the underlying frailty that allowed such a small setback to lead to death.

The high-wire metaphor illuminates the new importance of multiple coexisting serious illnesses and multiple competing causes of death. Some people will succumb to medical complications within a short time; others in a generally stable but fragile condition will evade fatal complications for a long time. Care that meets the needs of persons with serious, progressive chronic illness in the last phase of life will often have to be available to these individuals for many years. Some will use it that long, while others, who are no more seriously ill, will encounter their final complication and die much earlier. We cannot tell how long most people will have to live once they are living in a delicate balance with a fatal chronic condition.

Shortcomings in Current Care

Surgery, pacemakers, and intravenous antibiotics are readily available in the United States to most patients who need them while living with fatal chronic illness. Those in need generally have adequate insurance because they are old enough for Medicare, have private insurance through employment, or are poor enough for Medicaid. But few patients facing old age and eventually fatal chronic illnesses can count on some other essential elements of good care: for example, relief of symptoms, continuity of services and providers, a safe and functional environment, and help with planning for the future (Institute of Medicine 1997; Wenger et al. 2003).

The health-care system regularly fails to provide sufficient prevention and relief of pain. Among people living in nursing homes, one-fourth of those with pain every day received no pain medication at all, and another half had orders only for trivial kinds and amounts of medication (Bernabei et al. 1998). Another study showed that, among out-patients with pain from metastatic cancer, 42 percent did not receive adequate pain medication (Cleeland et al. 1994). Medications have proven effective in treating and managing pain, making it unnecessary—and even outrageous—for anyone to suffer from overwhelming pain or discomfort (National Cancer Policy Board 2001; Doyle, Hanks, and MacDonald 1998).

If a person's heart stops, a set of procedures called cardiopulmonary resuscitation (CPR) can sometimes get it started and the person's life can go on. A person with a sudden heart attack or injury ordinarily wants CPR tried, even though surviving it will usually mean living through a period of critical illness. However, a person with serious illness, disability, and short life expectancy may well prefer to forego attempts at CPR, accepting death when the heart stops rather than endure more travail for a small chance of a short, and even more disabled, survival. Good practice requires giving the patient (or a surrogate if the patient is too sick or otherwise unable to make decisions) the opportunity to consider the merits in advance and to decide whether CPR should be attempted. This seems obvious, yet a study of ten thousand patients hospitalized for at least a week with very advanced stages of serious illnesses found that doctors addressed this issue in less than half the cases (SUPPORT Principal Investigators 1995).

What each of us wants when close to the end of life is confidence that care will be there when we need it, that the people providing care will be competent and kind, and that we will have comfort and respect, right up to the end. But physicians now cannot promise patients with lung cancer or emphysema and facing a long course to death that every health-care provider in the area—every emergency room, nursing home, home-care agency, and hospice—is reliably competent to provide relief of pain and shortness of breath (National Cancer Policy Board 2001; Lynn and Goldstein 2003). Americans who face serious, eventually fatal, chronic illness must navigate a care system—really, a patchwork of uncoordinated services—that does not meet their needs and can even cause them harm (Institute of Medicine 2001). Furthermore, the costs of that care have increased substantially; for example, more than half of personal bankruptcy cases arise from health-care costs (Jacoby, Sullivan, and Warren 2001).

The Baby Boom Grows Old

The current population of thirty-five million Americans age sixty-five and older will more than double within the next thirty years (Federal Interagency Forum on Aging 2000). Indeed, the population's average age is increasing because women are having fewer babies and people are living twenty years longer than they did in 1950 (United Nations 2002). Additionally, the years after World War II saw a surge in births, and those babies are now aging (Kinsella and Velkoff 2001). The last century's baby boomers will be old enough to start having high rates of late-life disability between 2020 and 2030.

In the 1960s, when Medicare started, only 9 percent (seventeen million) of the population was sixty-five or older, and only 0.5 percent (one million) of the population was older than age eighty-five. In 2000, 12 percent (thirty-five million) of the population was sixty-five and older, and 1.5 percent (four million) was older than eighty-five. While the numbers of elderly persons will continue to rise, the major increase in serious disability will come when the baby-boom generation starts turning eighty-five in about 2030, when 22 percent of Americans (eighty million) will be over sixty-five, and 2.5 percent (nine million) will be over eighty-five (U.S. Census Bureau 2000).

The effects of the changing demographics will be stunning. Housing will need to accommodate wheelchairs and walkers, income support for retirement will have to last longer, and family and community organizations will have to make room for large numbers of persons with problems in mobility, hearing, vision, communication, and cognition. The services needed during the last few years of life are expensive. In fiscal year 2000, Medicaid paid for 45 percent of the $137 billion annual cost of institutional long-term care (U.S. Congress 2002). The Congressional Budget Office forecasts that the cost of long-term care will reach $207 billion in 2020 and $346 billion in 2040 (Congressional Budget Office 1999). These extraordinary costs risk bankrupting state budgets, which currently devote 20 percent of expenditures to Medicaid, while spending on all of health care constitutes about 30 percent of state spending (National Association of State Budget Officers 2003).

According to U.S. Senator John Breaux (D-LA, ranking member of the Senate Special Committee on Aging), "[Medicaid] has become our country's 'de facto' payer of long-term care for the elderly and disabled. Most people do not know Medicaid expenditures are now outpacing Medicare nor do they realize that Medicaid is the second largest expenditure for state budgets. The unsettling notion here is that we have no real, comprehensive long-term-care system in this country and yet we are spending billions of dollars for a system that was not designed—it just evolved. Unfortunately, the system we have is inefficient, outdated, incomplete and unable to meet the needs of current or future recipients" (Breaux 2002).

People worry that living longer will mean more disability and greater burdens on society. The jury is still out as to the actual aggregate effects. Several recent studies have documented an apparent reduction in the rate of serious disability in old age (Liao et al. 2000; Crimmins, Saito, and Reynolds 1997; Manton and Gu 2001). The studies are methodologically complex and the rate's reduction, if any, is slight (Lynn 2000; Freedman, Martin, and Schoeni 2002). Of course, some conditions, like arthritis, hearing and vision deficits, and dental decay, can often be prevented or delayed. However, if general frailty remains as the path to death in advanced old age, most people who live into advanced old age will inevitably endure substantial periods of serious disability before dying.

Fifty years ago, the United States had to build new schools, houses, hospitals, and sports facilities to accommodate a dramatic increase in the number of births: the baby boomers were here. As those boomers reach retirement, they present a similar problem: we do not have the facilities or resources to care for these aging people, especially when they are sick and dying. Five decades ago, we invested in schools and housing to meet the needs of a growing generation; today, we must invest in services to ensure appropriate and high-quality care for that generation as its members grow old and die.

Who Will Provide Care?

Living out the last years of life with serious chronic illness poses challenges that simply did not arise when people died quickly from heart attacks, pneumonias, childbirth infections, or influenza epidemics. Most people living with serious, progressive chronic illness need some other person's help just to get through the day, often every day, and sometimes constantly.

Unfortunately, our health-care and social systems have not yet fully recognized or begun to prepare for the upcoming frequency and extent of caregiving that the aged boomers will require. Indeed, most Americans have not absorbed the eventuality of needing to provide care for loved ones, and then needing it for themselves. Few people make plans to anticipate that sequence.

Foremost is the challenge of meeting the needs for hands-on personal care. Since most older people prefer to live in their own home or with family for as long as possible, both family and paid in-home caregivers are essential (McCorkle and Pasacreta 2001; Abel 1990; Koffman and Snow 2001; Ferrell 1998). Unpaid family caregiving has always been the backbone of long-term care. In a national random survey of adults in 2000, more than one-quarter stated that they had provided care for a chronically ill, disabled, or aged family member or friend in the past year. That translates into more than 50 million volunteer caregivers (National Family Caregivers Association 2000a). The federal Administration on Aging estimated that at any one time 22.4 million persons are providing family care (Administration on Aging 2003).

For married elders, the first one to develop an eventually fatal chronic illness can usually rely on the spouse for most of the direct care needed. In a study of all caregivers assisting people age sixty-five and older, spouses accounted for 24 percent, daughters for 20 percent, and sons for 6 percent, meaning that immediate family members are 50 percent of all caregivers (Kassner and Bectel 1998). The onset of illness in the caregiving spouse or in a widowed or unmarried elder often precipitates a crisis for the rest of the family, especially for the daughters and daughters-in-law, who most often assume the role of caregiver (Kassner and Bechtel 1998). Greater opportunities for women today in education and the workforce leave fewer unpaid workers for family care. Smaller family size and higher divorce rates also leave a smaller group of potential family caregivers (Noelker 2001). Single elderly people, whether widows, widowers, or unmarried, often must rely upon paid services (Tennstedt 1999). Even when children can pitch in to help with care, the need for paid help remains substantial (National Family Caregivers Association 2000a).

While most people who provide care to a family member do so out of loyalty and love, and most find it meaningful, the challenges of family caregiving are weighty (Assistant Secretary for Planning and Evaluation and Administration on Aging 1998). Depending on the family member's situation and health problem, family caregivers can assist with daily living tasks, with monitoring symptoms and general health, with administrating medications, and with coordinating care among health and social service providers, as well as with providing emotional support (Biegel, Sales, and Schulz 1991; Vitaliano 1997). The care system that a caregiver must negotiate is maddening in its lack of coordination and coherence. The average caregiving load is eighteen hours of direct services per week. Those providing care for persons who need help in at least two or more activities of daily living (activities like moving around, going to the toilet, or feeding and dressing oneself) average forty hours per week (National Alliance for Caregiving and the American Association of Retired Persons 1997). The majority of these caregivers hold paying jobs also, though one-third of those have incomes near the poverty line (Rigoglioso 2000). Two-thirds of family caregivers report that caregiving responsibilities have required that they rearrange work schedules, work fewer hours, or take unpaid leaves of absence. In addition, caregiving work can—and does—cause health problems for the caregiver (Schulz and Beach 1999; Kiecolt-Glaser et al. 1996). The average unpaid family caregiver is sixty years old. In a study of caregivers in New York City, 80 percent of the family caregivers had a serious chronic health problem themselves, and half had been caregivers for more than five years (Levine et al. 2000).

What has changed to make caregiving to the elderly a major challenge, when it seemed natural in the past?

First, reliance on family and friends a century ago was intense but brief; people were simply unlikely to live long with any severe disability. Now, family members have to give up work, rearrange households, and change their life plans for an indefinite—and often lengthy—time. The fragility of the ill person's life often calls for all manner of assiduous care, such as frequent cleanings, medications, feedings, and exercises. When medical issues arise, treatments often keep the patient alive but require even more intensive caregiving—doctor's visits, medications, hospitalizations, and visits to therapists. This intensive caregiving can go on for many years.

Second, in those "old days," the few disabled persons living through the last part of life had many descendants to rely upon. They might well be sole grandparents within large extended families. Now, the ratio of disabled elderly to their progeny is much smaller because family size has dropped at the same time that more elderly survive longer (Himes 1992). By 2020, an estimated 1.2 million people age sixty-five or older will have no living children, siblings, or spouses (National Aging Information Center 1996). In 1990, for each person over eighty-five years old, twenty-one people were between fifty and sixty-four; in 2030, only six will be in those prime caregiving years (Institute for Health and Aging 1996).

Third, today's potential caregivers ordinarily work outside the home, unless they have become ill and disabled themselves. When a woman took in a family member a century ago, she was already working at home. Now, she may have to give up her own income or accept less pay or advancement, if she herself is young enough to be employed and healthy enough to take on the hard work that elder care often requires. Since a family member who needs help at ninety-two years of age may have children who are past seventy, the nearest kin often already have their own health problems. Thus, an arrangement that was once fairly natural and routine now poses a real family crisis.

Fourth, the workforce for paid home health aides and home-care nurses has been shrinking. Once, home-care nursing was one of the few avenues for steady employment for poorly educated or otherwise unskilled women. Many immigrants found home nursing to be a way to have a safe abode and an income. It is, however, very hard work, often with difficult relationships and serious language barriers. Home care rarely offers health insurance, vacations, or other employee benefits. In addition, immigrating is harder, especially for those with few skills. The shortage of home health aides, combined with the problems in family caregiving, means that not enough hands will be available to provide all of the needed bed baths, feedings, or supervision. Increasing the availability of paid personnel to provide care may well require engendering career ladders, reasonable working conditions, and living wages—all of which entail costs (Rimer 2000).

Family caregiving has its costs too. As Senator Hillary Rodham Clinton has said, "Just because family caregiving is unpaid does not mean it is costless" (Lynch Schuster 2002). Indeed, the price tag on replacing family caregiving would be remarkably high: Arno and colleagues estimated its market value at $196 billion annually (Arno, Levine, and Memmott 1999). The costs to the family are only beginning to be understood. The daughter or daughter-in-law who up-ends her nuclear family's lives in order to provide for her parent or parent-in-law might be appreciated within the family, but she is also often forgotten by neighbors, churchgoers, friends, and employers. She gets a reduced pension and Social Security, risks going without health insurance, and has no disability protection. Because gender and caregiving limit women's savings and pensions, new-onset poverty in old age may largely affect women (Employee Benefit Research Institute 2002; Older Women's League 2004). Women now spend as long in caregiving for adult family members as in caring for children (Hooyman and Kiyak 1996). Nevertheless, women relatives continue to provide most of the hands-on care, with substantial variation by factors such as age, ethnic background, and proximity of family members.

Several studies have demonstrated the devastating effects of living with or caring for someone with a serious chronic illness. One-third of the families of hospitalized patients with serious illness lost most or all of their savings (Covinsky et al. 1994). The financial burden reflects not just the need to pay for medical services but also the lack of wages and benefits while providing care. In one study, family caregivers lost about $650,000 on average over a lifetime, considering wages, Social Security, and pension benefits (Metropolitan Life Insurance Company 1999).

One strategy would be to turn to paid caregivers. Paid vocational workers (not registered nurses) provide more than three-quarters of care in nursing homes and more than nine-tenths of paid care at home (Atchley 1996). By 2010, when the first baby boomers reach old age, the pool of middle-aged women available to provide low-skilled basic services will be substantially smaller than it is now (Feldman 1997). With pay scales barely above minimum wage for very difficult work, and with little or no health-care or disability insurance, few people find this line of work economically attractive (Himmelstein, Lewontin, and Woolhandler 1996; Wilner 2000). Citizens for Long-Term Care advocates such obvious workplace improvements as a living wage, a safe workload, adequate training, career opportunities, and employee supports such as child care and transportation (Citizens for Long-Term Care 2003). These demands, of course, have been part of industrial workers' contracts for many decades. A report to Congress from the Department of Health and Human Services and the Department of Labor reiterated these needs, framed by the recognition that, by conservative estimates, the United States will need three times as many paid long-term-care workers in 2050 as we will have in 2010 (U.S. Department of Health and Human Services and Department of Labor 2003).

In addition, the United States is in the midst of a shortage of nurses that will intensify as the baby boomers age and the need for health care grows. According to a July 2002 report, forty-four states plus the District of Columbia will have registered nurse shortages by the year 2020 (Health Resources and Services Administration 2003). More than one million new nurses will be needed by 2010 (U.S. Bureau of Labor Statistics 2001). Yet the number of first-time U.S.-educated nursing school graduates who sat for the national licensure examination for registered nurses fell by 25 percent between 1995 and 2002 (National Council of State Boards of Nursing 2002). Moreover, 75 percent of all hospitals have vacancies for nurses already (American Hospital Association 2001).

Whereas other nations provide payment, respite, tax breaks, training, and other support for family caregivers, the United States generally does not. Under Germany's plan, for example, patients requiring long-term care can choose between the formal care system and a cash payout, which allows them to pay family members who provide assistance. In addition, these paid family caregivers receive pension credit and qualify for respite services (Noelker 2001). The United States does have a limited demonstration project like this, called Cash and Counseling. Generally, though, the United States provides almost no regular or reliable support to family or paid caregivers who serve patients with eventually fatal chronic illness. While finding the financial and structural resources to care for large numbers of disabled elderly in 2020 will be challenging on many fronts, the coming shortage of persons able and willing to provide hands-on care appears to be the most implacable challenge.

"Dying" and the Problem of Prognostication

After the writings of Elizabeth Kübler-Ross (1969) and the ensuing wave of attention popularized the term, "dying" came to connote a period of rapid, progressive illness and disability after treatment failed. Family and caregivers—indeed, patients themselves—learned to expect that "dying" individuals would put their affairs in order and be dead within a very short time, no more than a month or two. A physician could label a patient with weight loss, weakness, and metastatic cancer, for example, as "dying." That label triggered a pattern of behaviors for patient, family, and clinicians. Friends expected the "dying" person to go through "stages" of dying (denial, anger, bargaining, and acceptance) in about that order (Kübler-Ross 1969). Family and friends assumed that "dying" people would not make long-term plans or pursue long-shot therapies but would instead make peace with the ending of their lives and say their good-byes to loved ones.

Among the major causes of death, only cancer routinely has a confined period of time, usually less than eight weeks, in which the patient loses weight, energy, and ability to carry on daily tasks (McCarthy et al. 2000; Morris et al. 1986). Such a patient discontinues most activities, often asks for increased comfort care, and ordinarily dies at a rather predictable time. But only about one-quarter of all deaths are from cancer (National

Center for Health Statistics 2001), and most serious chronic illnesses follow a very different course. The relatively quick and predictable course of dying with cancer is no longer the only useful model around which to organize medical care or social supports.

Most Americans die with failure of a major organ (heart, lungs, kidneys, or liver), dementia, stroke, or general frailty of old age (Murphy 2000; Lunney 2000; Lunney et al. 2003). Unlike cancer, these conditions lead to long periods of diminished function and involve multiple unpredictable and serious exacerbations of symptoms. The timing of death for individuals with these diseases is ordinarily not predictable. And unless their course mimics that of terminal cancer—with a discernable period of rapidly declining weight, strength, and function—people with these less predictable diseases cannot be classified as "dying." If they never have such a phase, then death comes unexpectedly and without preparations. They do not qualify for hospice or have plans to avoid resuscitation. In short, while patients die from heart failure or emphysema, for example, they often do so with no discernable phase that can be labeled "dying."

I have often heard a family member of one of my patient say something like, "If I had only known Mother was dying, I would have come home to be with her." The mother had been on oxygen for many months and was over ninety years old. Surely, I would think, this seventy-year-old person could not have expected his or her mother to go on forever. Yet the survivor assumed that there would be a time of "dying," a time for good-byes, and regretted missing that opportunity.

The degree to which the timing of death is not predictable is surprising to the public. Somehow, most of us have the sense that physicians could tell us how much time we have left, if they wanted to (and if we asked). One project studied the medical records of nearly ten thousand seriously ill patients; interviewed the patients, family members, and physicians; and then developed a set of mathematical formulas that predict the timing of death (Knaus et al. 1995). For one hundred people with a particular disease, the predictive formulas were quite accurate. If the predictions said that half would die within six months, about half actually died by then. Asking physicians to make predictions about their own patients yielded about the same good average accuracy. But neither approach worked very well to predict the timing of death for a specific patient. Substantially erroneous predictions in optimistic or pessimistic directions average out for groups but scramble the reliability for individuals.

Figure 1 reflects the striking unreliability of predictions for persons who turn out to be very near death. Even in the last weeks of life, many patients have good odds of living another two months. Lung cancer (here, "non-small-cell" inoperable cancer that started in the lung) is one of the most predictable among fatal conditions. Once the person is seriously ill and losing weight, survival for more than a few weeks becomes quite unlikely. Nevertheless, just seven days before dying, the median patient with lung cancer still has almost a 50–50 chance of living for two months. How can that be? It turns out that a substantial number of lung cancer patients have their course cut short by a complication—an infection, a bad reaction to treatment, a heart attack, or something else that crops up unpredictably and shortens life. In each case, the physicians and the patients and families all knew that the patients had fatal lung cancer, but just a few days before death, no one could know that life would end this week. All involved might say, "But he didn't really die of his cancer; this complication was what caused his death." Without his cancer, of course, the complication would have been unlikely to prove fatal.

Heart failure death is much less predictable than lung cancer death. All of the heart failure patients in this study were very ill. They had been in the hospital with shortness of breath, they were on multiple medications to boost circulation and protect the heart, and they were unable to walk far or to climb stairs. They clearly would die of their heart failure, unless something even worse came along. They would have long periods of stable function, too. They would come home from the hospital and get settled, figure out how to avoid having to climb steps or carry groceries, and live fairly well for some time. Then some complication would arise, often from a relatively small thing like having a cold or eating too much salt; and the delicate balance would tip over into a serious struggle to breathe.

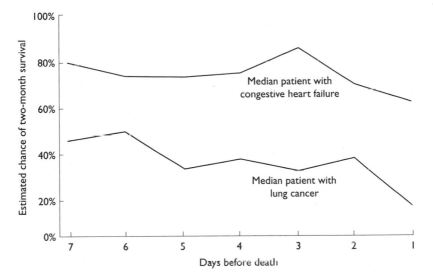

Figure 1.   Predicted likelihood of two-month survival, several days before death from heart failure or lung cancer. Source: Lynn, Harrell, et al. 1996.

Hospital care would generally pull the person through, more than once. Eventually, though, one of these episodes would prove fatal, or the damaged heart would simply lose its regular rhythm and fail to pump. Either way, the death most often happened within a week of the patient having been stable, though living with serious constraints on activity.

When asked to predict timing of death for persons who are very sick, physicians usually give estimates that are a bit generous (Christakis 1999). The reasons for this are unclear, but wishing to be kind or to avoid anger from patients and families who make plans around the prediction may well play a role. One study asked physicians to state a likelihood of the patient surviving for two or for six months; and that question, on average, got accurate answers (Zhong and Lynn 1999). So the answers physicians give may depend somewhat on the question asked.

Since the timing of death for individual patients is usually unpredictable, in order to provide reliably good care in the last phase of life, the care system will have to be able to deliver good care to some people for years, not just for the last weeks or months. Building a set of desirable services that is available only to those who are sure to die soon is not a strategy that would actually include most dying people.

Nevertheless, that is exactly what the Medicare hospice benefit aimed to do. Hospice (which I discuss in chapter 3) is an effective provider of comprehensive end-of-life services, mostly to persons dying at home. The Medicare hospice benefit requires the attending physician to certify that the patient has a prognosis of less than six months. Remarkably, the federal regulation has never specified whether that prognosis should be "virtually certain" or just "more likely than not" (Lynn 2001). Obviously, it is a very different thing to predict anything with certainty than it is to bet the odds. On the one hand, allowing the "more likely than not" definition acknowledges the uncertainty of individual predictions but also means that many people will qualify for hospice care throughout many months, even years. Those will be the people whose luck held out; they walked a long time on the high wire before encountering their final complication. On the other hand, adopting a "virtually certain to die" definition means that hospice will be available to a much smaller cohort, mostly very near death, and dying of conditions that allow prediction, at least when death is coming very soon. Hospice enrollment patterns and the government's audits for fraud seem to use mostly a definition of prognostic eligibility that is closer to "virtually certain to die" than to "more likely than not." Hence most people die from serious chronic disease and never have the opportunity to use hospice, since they went from an ambiguous prognosis to death within a few days.

The impact of these observations is just beginning to shape the thinking of professionals and the public. Whereas once the family doctor told the anguished parents of a child with diphtheria or whooping cough that the child would get better or die within a few days, now patients ask, "How long do I have?" and doctors are often inarticulate about why they cannot readily answer the question. It turns out that most of us now die with unpredictable timing from predictably fatal chronic disease. The fact that the condition will eventually be fatal is clear, and the survival statistics for a large group of affected patients may likewise be clear, but a reliable prediction for one patient is not possible. Two patients with the same amount of heart damage and the same array of concurrent illnesses might have very different life spans for largely unpredictable reasons. Dying "suddenly" in the midst of long-term chronic conditions is a common pattern for the end of life. But we have not yet learned a set of metaphors and expressions that gives voice to that experience, and we certainly have not yet learned how best to live and die in this situation.

Which Illness Will It Be?

Our national priorities in health care are said to be "to promote health and quality of life by preventing and controlling disease, injury, and disability" (Centers for Disease Control and Prevention 2002a). The headlines trumpeting a success often say something like "New Drug Promises to Save 10,000 Lives per Year," or "Treatment Offers Hope to Millions." "Saving lives" and "offering hope" are metaphors brought forward from the triumphs of public health in the past century, when millions of children actually did live full lives rather than dying from polio or diphtheria.

What is missing is the recognition that opportunities for prevention and treatment eventually run up against mortality. Immunizing a town's children to save them from polio has obvious benefits in terms of extended life duration and life opportunities. Saving a young adult from death from meningitis with a few doses of antibiotics generates the same enthusiasm. Yet saving a frail nursing-home resident from any particular complication extends life a bit, changes the manner of dying, and may or may not, on balance, be a good thing (Rich and Sox 2000; Lynn and Cretin 2000). When we use the language of prevention and cure, we often carry along the enthusiasm and approval from historical triumphs of public health and medical treatment, but these sentiments may not fit the current situation.

When public health aims at "preventing and controlling disease, injury and disability," it tries to reduce the incidence (the rate of new cases) and prevalence (the rate in the population at any one time) of disease and disability. Among very sick or very old people, these measures are inadequate and possibly misleading. Most people living their last few years now have multiple medical problems—co-morbidities, to use technical language—from diseases or just from old age. Preventing one condition from causing illness and death necessarily means increasing the likelihood that another one will cause illness and death, just a little later (Welch et al. 1996). If a person has some heart disease and some memory problems, as well as the reduced reserves of all of the organs that come with being eighty-eight years old, then treatments that slow the heart problem will increase the chances that the person will live long enough to be greatly burdened by memory problems. Again, that may or may not be desirable.

People would expect a headline that shouts "New Drug Prevents Heart Disease in Elderly" to herald a story about something thoroughly laudable. The headline could be equally correct and say instead "New Drug Promises Major Increases in Dementia." Saving the lives of children who otherwise faced polio was reasonably understood to be a very good thing. Saving the lives of elderly persons by eliminating one among a group of competing causes of death is more complicated. Eliminating one illness might well change the nature of the death and delay its timing, but the language of saving lives is misleading.

Half of the elderly who survive one trip to an intensive-care unit die within a year (Rockwood et al. 1993). By age eighty-five, most people have more than two established diagnoses of conditions that can be expected to worsen and cause death (Wolff, Starfield, and Anderson 2002). A quarter century ago, Tauber (1976) computed the effects of eliminating cancer as a cause of death and found less than a year of prolonged survival on average (and a substantial increase in the likelihood of dying from heart disease). Winning the war against a particular cancer would yield major gains for a few people who now die young, but it would mostly have small effects on older people, since old age is when most people die of cancer. Another illness is, all too often, waiting in the wings.

Welch and colleagues (1996) pointed out that the expected mortality risk for a patient was composed of the risks associated with aging and the risks associated with particular conditions. Thus, a young person's risk of dying with a medical condition almost entirely arises from the risks associated with that condition alone, since the risks associated with aging are slight. However, an older person faces substantial risks from an array of aging-associated illnesses. Indeed, those risks can greatly attenuate the merits of treating any one specific disease. For example, mild prostate cancer can have a 5 percent mortality at five years. A sixty-five-year-old man will lose an average of two years to that disease, changing his predicted survival from fifteen years to thirteen years. The same cancer in an eighty-five year-old will cost him only a few months on average, shaved off his expected survival for five years.

The age-related component of a patient's mortality risk becomes much more substantial with increasing age, so the contribution of successful treatment or prevention of any particular illness becomes correspondingly smaller. In addition, older persons usually have more burdens and more limited success from interventions, considerations that further limit the merits of intervening. Of course, estimates of future survival and function should consider the patient's actual condition, not just the patient's age; and age-related risks apply to predicting disability as well as mortality. The upshot is that, for persons approaching the end of life, it is common to find that treatment is not worth its burdens. If a person is living with one fatal illness and evidences another, very often the suffering imposed by treatment more than outweighs the possible advantage of success in that treatment.

None of these outcomes argue against prevention or cure. Our success in meeting those aims gives us the opportunity to live long before becoming mortally ill. Even in advanced illness and old age, some conditions merit prevention or cure: pain or skin ulcers, for example. But

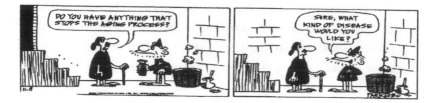

Figure 2. Ultimate options. Reprinted by permission of John L. Hart, FLP, and Creators Syndicate, Inc.

there is no way to avoid aging, really, except to die young (figure 2). Exercise, good diet, mammograms, and colonoscopies help delay the onset of serious illness, but each person's future includes a fatal condition.

Now that Americans mostly live into old age before becoming seriously burdened with chronic illness, we need more appropriate language and metaphors. We hope to live as well as possible, even with serious illness. It matters to ease symptoms, enhance autonomy, avoid bankruptcy, alleviate depression, and otherwise relieve what suffering can be relieved, even in the "valley of the shadow of death." But we can't tackle these urgent issues unless we learn to reach beyond the folly of focusing only on prevention and cure.

Costs and Who Pays

Most people who are sick enough to die have insurance coverage. More than four-fifths have Medicare (Hogan et al. 2000). Another group has veterans' benefits or employer-sponsored insurance. Those who have lived in poverty, or who become impoverished as part of their illness, qualify for Medicaid. Among the rest, probably half die relatively young and quickly from infections, accidents, and violence. So no more than a tenth die of serious chronic illness in conventional employer-sponsored insurance or without insurance. Federal funding and regulation dominate care for serious chronic illness in America.

The real costs of care are hard to calculate. Medicare's payments average about $28,000 in the last year of a person's life (Emanuel et al. 2002). Given that Medicare now pays about half of the costs (Maxwell, Moon, and Segal 2001; Lubitz et al. 2003), the average total cost is around $50,000 for the last year of life. Private payments or Medicaid, not Medicare, cover most of nursing-home care, long-term paid support at home, and prescription drugs. On average, people now are seriously ill for much more than one year (Lynn, Blanchard, et al. 2002). Two years is probably the average for self-care disability, but some are disabled for more than a decade. Compared to younger people, older Medicaid beneficiaries use less medical and hospital treatment as they die but more long-term care (Scitovsky 1988).

Medicare spends about half as much for the last year of life for people dying past ninety years old as for those sixty-five to seventy-five (Bird, Shugarman, and Lynn 2002). Yet it spends comparatively more for the second and third years before older people's death (Shugarman et al. 2004). Older patients are disabled longer and their end-of-life expenditures are lower per year, but their illnesses often continue for years (Spillman and Lubitz 2000; Lubitz and Riley 1993). Hence people who die at seventy-three and ninety-three, for example, cost Medicare nearly the same amount (Lubitz et al. 2003).

While costs earlier in life show substantial disparities, Medicare's costs for the last year of life average almost the same for the poor and the rich, for blacks and whites, for women and men, and for people dying of stroke, heart failure, emphysema, or cancer (Shugarman et al. 2004). Since substantial disparities affect most of health care (Collins et al. 2002), that last year of life is a surprising leveler. Age continues to be a substantial factor, as outlined earlier. Geography also shapes expenses (Dartmouth Atlas of Health Care 1998), with much lower costs in Oregon than in New York, for example.

Medicare's costs for the last year of life have been stable at about 26 percent of the program budget for two decades (Hoover et al. 2002). The costs per capita for Medicare have increased, even when adjusted for inflation, but the costs in the last year of life are no different from any others in this regard (Barnato et al. 2004). Population growth, population aging, and added coverage for those with disabilities, end-stage renal failure, and amyotrophic lateral sclerosis (or Lou Gehrig's disease) have increased the number of people in Medicare from under twenty million in 1966, as the program got under way, to over forty million in 2002 (U.S. Department of Health and Human Services 2003).

As many analyses have found, payments for Medicare-covered services in any given year are highly concentrated among a small number of beneficiaries who have multiple chronic conditions and whose medical care is extremely expensive (Hogan et al. 2000; Crippen 2002). While end-of-life costs have remained stable as a proportion of Medicare outlays over time (Lubitz and Riley 1993; Hogan et al. 2000), Medicare payments for the last year of life averaged about $28,000, six times the per capita cost for survivors. The costliest 5 percent of beneficiaries consumed about half of total Medicare spending, and the costliest 25 percent consumed almost 90 percent. While such beneficiaries are more likely to die than the average beneficiary, many of those who live continue to have high costs in later years as a result of chronic medical conditions. About 84 percent of all Medicare beneficiaries have at least one chronic condition, and 62 percent have two or more chronic conditions (Anderson, Horvath, and Anderson 2002). Long-term-care expenditures for older U.S. residents with disabilities (including those receiving nursing-home or community-based care) totaled $123 billion in 2000, with more than 65 percent paid by the government (Crippen 2002).

Of the $1.2 trillion spent in 2001 on personal health care, about $0.1 trillion went to nursing-home care (Walker 2002), and $0.9 trillion went to the noninstitutional care of those with chronic conditions (Anderson, Horvath, and Anderson 2002). In constant dollars, these expenditures were expected to double before 2040, even without the inclusion of prescription drugs in Medicare in 2003 (Hoffman and Rice 1995, 9).

Long-term-care services have become an important part of health-care costs, growing from 3.3 percent in 1960 to 10.8 percent in 1995

(Employee Benefit Research Institute 1997). Funds come from a combination of sources, which include federal, state, local, private insurance, and out-of-pocket. Approximately $137 billion was spent in 2000 on long-term care (Walker 2002), with 37 percent coming from patients and families (without including the costs for unpaid family caregivers or wages lost because of caregiving). Medicaid pays for about half of institutional long-term care (Stone 2002).

A recent estimate of total lifetime health-care costs from multiple data sources shows that half of all expenditures occur past age 65; and for those who live to age 85, more than one-third of costs are incurred in remaining years (Alemayehu and Warner 2004). As the authors point out, these data starkly illuminate the challenge of growing numbers of older Americans.

The Shape of Things to Come

A major success of modern medical care is that we will be fairly healthy through most of life. But eventually, the facts of mortality will catch each of us—author, readers, general public. And for most of us, eventually fatal chronic illness generates the most substantial expense and, perhaps, the most unexamined challenge we face.

No one can count on good care. Some combination of pain, disability, financial ruin, family stress, and powerlessness awaits most of us. We could let it drift and just hope for good luck; but we could do better, so much better. We all have a stake in this, for ourselves and those we love, and for the community at large. At least for the next half century, more and more of us will be coming to the end of life together—doubling the annual number over the next two decades. The outlines of effective reforms are becoming clear, and the case for them is becoming compelling.

The Loneliness of the Long-Term Care Giver
Carol Levine

On the icy morning of January 15, 1990, my husband lay comatose in the emergency room of a community hospital after an automobile accident. . . . My husband did survive. . . . But he will never walk, and he is not the same person in any sense. . . .

Although I worried most about his mental functioning, it is his body that has recovered least. He is totally disabled and requires 24-hour care. He is incontinent of bladder and bowel. He is quadriparetic, with mobility limited to the partial use of his left hand. (His right forearm was amputated. . . .)

During my nine-year odyssey, I stopped being a wife and became a family care giver. In the anxious weeks when my husband was in the intensive care unit, I was still a wife. Doctors and nurses informed me of each day's progress or setbacks and treated me with kindness and concern. At some point, however, when he was no longer in immediate danger of dying, and as the specialists and superspecialists drifted out of the picture, I became invisible. Then, when the devastating and permanent extent of his disabilities became clear to clinicians, I became visible again.

At that point, I was important only as the manager and, it was expected, the hands-on provider of my husband's care. In retrospect, I date my rite of passage into the role of family care giver to the first day of my husband's stay in a rehabilitation facility, a place I now think of as a boot camp for care givers. A nurse stuck my husband's soiled sweat pants under my nose and said, "Take these away. Laundry is your job.". . . The nurse's underlying message, reinforced by many others, was that my life from now on would consist of performing an unrelieved series of nasty chores.

The social worker assigned to my husband's case had one goal: discharge. I was labeled a "selfish wife," since I refused to take him home without home care. "Get real," the social worker said. "Nobody will pay for home care. You have to quit your job and 'spend down' to get on Medicaid." . . .

When I brought my husband home, he had undiagnosed severe sleep apnea (which caused nighttime screaming), undiagnosed hearing loss, and poorly treated major depression. The first few months at home were nightmarish. Since the problems had not been diagnosed correctly, much less treated, I did not know where to turn. . . .

In addition to holding a full-time job, I manage all my husband's care and daily activities. Being a care manager requires grit and persistence. It took me 10 days of increasingly insistent phone calls to get my managed-care company to replace my husband's dangerously unstable hospital bed. When the new bed finally arrived—without notice, in the evening, when there was no aide available to move him—it turned out to be the cheapest model, unsuitable for a patient in my husband's condition. In these all-too-frequent situations, I feel that I am challenging Goliath with a tiny pebble. More often than not, Goliath just puts me on hold.

Being a care manager also takes money. I now pay for a daytime home care aide and serve as the night nurse myself. . . . Home care aides, disposable supplies, and most forms of therapy are not covered, because they are "not medically necessary." My husband recently needed a new customized wheelchair, which cost $3,700; the managed-care company paid $500. Medicare, his secondary payer, has so far rejected all claims. No one advocates on my husband's behalf except me; no one advocates on my behalf, not even me.

I feel abandoned by a health care system that commits resources and rewards to rescuing the injured and ill but then consigns such patients and their families to the black hole of chronic "custodial" care. . . .

Families need emotional support. They frequently bring a patient home to a living space transformed by medical equipment and a family life constrained by illness. Privacy is a luxury. Every day must be planned to the minute. The intricate web of carefully organized care can unravel with one phone call from an aide who is ill, an ambulette service that does not show up, a doctor's office that cannot accommodate a wheelchair, an equipment company that does not have an emergency service. There are generally no extra hands to help out in a crisis and no experienced colleagues to ask for advice. Friends and even family members fade away.

Excerpted with permission from Levine C. 1999. The loneliness of the long-term care giver. *N Engl J Med.* 340:1587–1590. Copyright © 1999 Massachusetts Medical Society. All rights reserved.

2

SEEING THE WORLD DIFFERENTLY

Ideas to Shape Reform

Facts are like geography—they shape the possibilities. Interpretations are like politics—they create the human structures and meanings. The facts of the last chapter shape the terrain and give rise to a number of possible interpretations and perspectives. This chapter will offer the interpretations that I have come to see as the most important in order to generate a reliable, sustainable set of social arrangements to support the last phase of life.

Life Span Perspective

A remarkable proportion of overall health-care needs and costs is now concentrated in the last few years of the life span. Most of the costs—and the burdens—of bad health arise with serious chronic illness in the last tenth of life. Figure 3 illustrates how experienced physicians and managers estimate the distribution of total health-care costs over the typical American's lifetime. Since no database records these expenses directly, expert estimates are our only source. Existing data strongly support the estimate for the last year of life. During that year, a Medicare beneficiary ordinarily uses more than $25,000 in health-care costs; the preceding two years add up to about the same total (Hogan et al. 2000; Shugarman et al. 2004). But we must double the sum of these last three years because Medicare covers only about half the costs (for example, Medicare does not cover

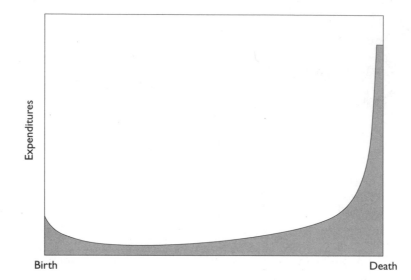

Figure 3.   Pattern of health-care expenditures across a person's life. The gray area under the curve equals all health-care expenditures over a typical life span. Source: Lynn and Adamson 2003.

nursing-home costs or prescription drugs) (Maxwell, Moon, and Segal 2001). Assuming an eighty-year life span, each tenth of the life span would be eight years. The costs of the last three years of life add up to around $100,000, and another $5,000 per year (close to average Medicare expenses) is a reasonable figure for the five years before. Thus, the last tenth of life incurs roughly $125,000 in health-care costs, probably nearly half of the costs over the person's lifetime. More reliable estimates would be well worth having, but the concentration of costs in the last part of life will be striking, even though neither the patients nor the clinicians may see those services as having anything to do with the end of life at the time they are provided (Alemayehu and Warner 2004).

A similar curve for the U.S. population in 1900 would have been much flatter, both because serious illnesses were more common throughout life and because death often occurred suddenly in the course of a generally healthy life. Moving the bulk of serious illness into old age is a laudable achievement. Even so, having a few years of serious disability at the close of life has become both commonplace and costly.

Rethinking the Transition Model

When Elisabeth Kübler-Ross sought to study "dying" people in the late 1960s, clinicians responded that her university hospital had no one known to be dying (Kübler-Ross 1969). To label some people as "dying" and tailor care for them in order to better serve them was a revolutionary idea to professionals and public alike. Indeed, that insight spurred the hospice movement. But, however comforting a split between "dying" and "not dying" is to those who feel themselves to be "not dying," the labels don't fit people very well. Chapter 1 showed that the boundary between being mortally ill and merely sick turns out to be hard to find or predict.

Policy makers and their public do not yet have language that adequately expresses the types of care individuals facing eventually fatal chronic illnesses need most. The language popularly associated with palliative care alludes to a turning away from conventional care (figure 4, top). If the model were correct that "dying" people are a discrete, easily distinguishable group, then patients would get "aggressive care" until that treatment became ineffective, when they would be "dying" and would turn to "palliative or hospice care," which included only symptomatic treatment.

But some patients need pain control early and disease-modifying treatments late. Thus, the lower diagram in figure 4 embodies a better concept, with the proportion of disease-modifying treatments (often wrongly called "curative"), declining and the proportion of palliative care increasing as a patient's condition worsens and the end of life comes closer. In addition, the improved model recognizes the family's need for support in bereavement.

Many in the health-care arena now talk about most end-of-life care as "palliative," or comfort, care, without really agreeing on a definition. The Last Acts Task Force defined palliative care as "the comprehensive

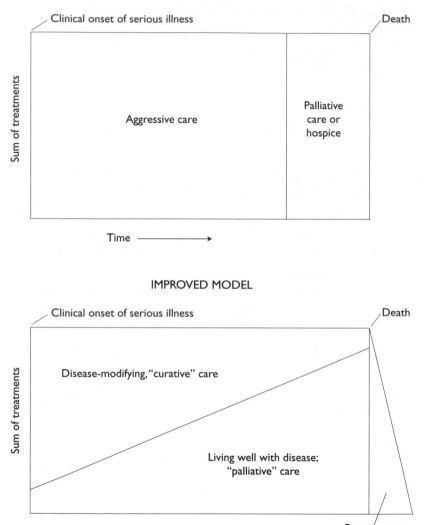

CONVENTIONAL MODEL

Clinical onset of serious illness

Death

Sum of treatments

Aggressive care

Palliative care or hospice

Time ⟶

IMPROVED MODEL

Clinical onset of serious illness

Death

Sum of treatments

Disease-modifying, "curative" care

Living well with disease; "palliative" care

Time ⟶

Bereavement

Figure 4. Appropriate care near the end of life. Source: Lynn and Adamson 2003.

management of the physical, psychological, social, spiritual and exis-
tential needs of patients" (Last Acts 1997), whereas the World Health
Organization defined it more narrowly as "the active total care of patients whose disease is not responsive to curative treatment" (World
Health Organization 1990). Last Acts' definition might reasonably
apply to patients at all stages of their illness—from diagnosis to death,
even while cure may still be likely. Indeed, it seems to encompass all care
services. The Center to Advance Palliative Care (www.capc.org) uses
the term generally for the bottom half of the lower diagram: palliative
services that are contemporaneous with services to modify the course of
the illness. Probably the definitions will converge in the next few years;
in the meantime, those who use the term may well have to define it as
they use it in order to avoid misunderstanding.

The upper diagram's pervasive mental model of a transition from one
kind of care to another works only if a patient really "turns a corner" for
the worse and the usual medical treatment clearly becomes futile, making all care thereafter palliative. For many patients, it will never be appropriate to "give up" all aggressive treatments (Byock 2000). Even
though they want to be as comfortable as possible, patients may choose
to have certain procedures or treatments that extend life. They want *some*
palliative care, but not *exclusively* palliative care (Selwyn and Forstein
2003).

For example, a person with emphysema may well want a trial of ventilator support for the next time his breathing gets seriously impaired;
but that same person might want advance care planning, a strict limit on
how long to try the ventilator, and the promise of sedation at the end
when the ventilator is withdrawn as he directed. Or someone with a
stroke might reasonably want aggressive treatment to reduce the chances
of another stroke and vigorous rehabilitation to enhance self-care potential, while also wanting strong measures for the pain associated with
contractures in the unused hand. In most medical situations, the goals of
living comfortably, independently, and longer are not in conflict, and,
quite reasonably, patients want them all.

Misleading Words and Ideas

The language that we commonly use to discuss illness, treatment, and payment is also becoming misleading. Ever since the Renaissance, people have identified illnesses first by giving a diagnosis. Indeed, for much of that time, providing a diagnosis was one of a physician's most important services. Even now, much of health care is organized by diagnosis. Each condition usually includes a wide range of stages, starting with minor problems and progressing to serious, advanced illness. The diagnosis alone does not tell much about severity. Furthermore, most of the people who are very sick and coming toward the end of life have more than one important diagnosis. Finally, diagnosis may not characterize needs well. Being unable to climb stairs means needing help in getting the groceries in, whether you have heart trouble or hip trouble; but many people with heart or hip trouble can climb steps. Being unable to think clearly or remember your situation requires supervision around the clock, whether the cognitive failure arose from strokes or Alzheimer's dementia.

Health-care delivery is organized by its setting—nursing home, hospital, home, and doctor's office. The setting governs how insurance pays bills, providers meet with patients, and regulations apply. However, patients with serious chronic illness change settings often. No longer is it enough to deliver high-quality hospital care for heart disease—the hospital's contribution to good outcomes means little if the next provider (such as a nursing home or physician's office) cannot play its role well. Patients, family members, and even policy makers will need to learn to assess performance with regard to the populations who are very sick and nearing the end of life in all their settings, rather than evaluating quality of care or costs only in particular care settings or with particular diagnoses or treatments. The scope of good care must include nursing homes, bed baths, advance care planning, and bereavement, as well as surgical operations, preventive services, and rehabilitation.

Some other commonplace terms also need remodeling. Statistics on the cause of death have shaped research and treatment priorities for years, and most people believe that this classification is as reliable and obvious as gender or age. Not true. When a person dies after trauma or sudden pneumonia at age fifty, it makes sense to say that this one problem was the cause of death. For most people now, the situation is much more complicated. First, the person is often sick enough and old enough that no one wants to put him or her through much travail to get a specific diagnosis, since no diagnosis could make a difference in treatment or outcome. Indeed, many people carry serious diagnoses that are never rigorously investigated and might well be misleading. In the very old, the rate of correct diagnoses of heart failure probably includes only about half of those who have had a medical bill for heart failure (Barnato et al. 2003). Sometimes, in contrast, the person carries a number of diagnoses, and which one "caused" death is difficult to discern. Even the doctor often cannot know exactly what combination of problems caused death. Autopsy would provide a great deal of information about the body's infirmities, but almost no expected deaths, especially in old age, give rise to autopsies (Podbregar et al. 2001).

Just as overall decline and multisystem failure in old age confound the diagnosis and cause of death, the very images of sickness, health, and dying come into question. Once, a person was healthy, then sick, and then usually either recovered or died within a few weeks. The classic outline of a physician-patient encounter assumes that the patient has a chief complaint, gets a diagnosis, and adopts a temporary "sick role," shedding usual responsibilities and roles in order to recover. In contrast, many patients now have many symptoms and problems, rather than a chief complaint, and the physician may find multiple well-established diagnoses, or no clear diagnosis at all, and still have to help patients cope with a difficult situation. The sick role is often lifelong and thus becomes normal life.

Again, this amounts to a new way of thinking. Instead of assuming that sick roles are part of the process of getting well, society must recognize that the natural course of life now includes living with a worsening degenerative disease in the last phase of life. As each person accumulates illnesses, risk factors, and loss of reserves, the balance of factors necessary for life becomes increasingly fragile. Smaller disruptions become enough to tip over the balance and make the person seriously ill. With that image in mind, symptoms and disabilities might be more important than diagnoses as we match patients with services. Rather than organizing payment and quality assessment by settings of care, we might do better to focus on the populations that need ongoing services as they move among multiple settings. Perhaps we could, more rationally, tie funding and regulation to the patients rather than to the setting for care. Furthermore, rather than linking resource allocation for care and research to "cause of death" statistics, our public priorities might reflect an effort to maximize comfort and capabilities as well as length of life.

Many opinion leaders have railed at the inadequacies of the acute-care model and have proposed various alternatives (Institute of Medicine 2001; Fox 1993; Wagner 1998). Oddly, the most prominent efforts to gain public attention for a chronic-care model hardly take note of the fact that serious chronic illness generally leads to death (see www.improvingchroniccare.org; www.nccconline.org). Major publications on prevalence and impact of chronic illness simply do not mention that the end of chronic illness is death or that the impact of chronic illness tends to become more pervasive and severe toward the end of life (Institute for Health and Aging 1996; Centers for Disease Control and Prevention 2002b). Chronic illness somehow pops up in the middle of a life, unconnected to its necessary end in death.

Disregard for death as the outcome of serious chronic illness is unfortunate, since the fact of implacable decline and death is important in shaping the patient's experience and judging the real merits of treatment strategies. Many elderly people would choose to have a care delivery system that made it harder to use hospitals, in return for having reliable help at home (Lynn, O'Connor, et al. 1999). An eighty-two-year-old with fragile health, for example, may well be a suitable candidate for heart surgery, but he may also reflect that his prostate cancer and his memory problems will continue to get worse and that the months of recuperation from surgery will ruin the best time he otherwise has left.

Thus, part of the work needed to undergird reform involves changes in perception. The categories of the past prevent our seeing current realities. Working with patterns of need as they change over time seems better than working only with diagnoses and settings of care. The time has come to abandon the expectation that patients will have a "transition from cure to care," to use the common phrase for changing the orientation of health care as the patient nears death. Often our mental models, categories, and language need updating in order to enable needed reforms.

The "No Surprise" Question

The data on prognosis show just how uncertain forecasting survival time often is. For a few decades, our society has given special attention to certain people because they are not expected to live long. As noted earlier, the category of "dying" marks people who are overwhelmingly likely to die within a few weeks, or maybe a month or two. It includes a strongly stereotyped set of behaviors about those who are terminally ill or "dying": friends and family are to visit, the patient is to say good-byes and bless the living, the care system is to be gentle and unobtrusive, and death is to come within the expected time. But a serious and pervasive inability to prognosticate with precision complicates this approach. For example, a person can have heart failure sufficient to have a life expectancy of less than six months and yet have a 5 percent chance of dying within a week or the same 5 percent likelihood of living for five years. Most people who die will not have a discernible period of terminal illness, but most will have been quite ill before death. If we allow special attention and behaviors only to those who are virtually sure to die soon, that minority will feel that they must conform, while everyone else will encounter resistance when they attend to their mortality.

Who should receive special services because they are at the end of life?

The only defensible category I have been able to find takes in people who are already very sick with a condition that is expected to cause death, even if they may live for many months or years. This cohort includes most of the people with serious illnesses in the last years of life but not many people who actually recover and do well thereafter for a substantial period of time.

Many clinical settings have found that a useful way to identify these patients is by asking their physicians and nurses: "Is this person sick enough that it would be no surprise if he or she died within the coming year (or the coming few months)?" (Lynn, Schall, et al. 2000; Lynn, Schuster, and Kabcenell 2000). It generally does not matter if the time frame is a few months or a year, since the issue is whether the current illness could worsen and cause the person's death. This "no surprise" question has worked well for targeting clinical improvement activities, though it has not been tested in regulatory, financing, or more formal service delivery innovations. Some patients identified in this way will die quickly and some will live a long time, but all are sick enough that they would benefit from comprehensive services tailored to advanced illness and the last part of life. Often, this question identifies patients who are "too sick" to come to see the doctor; they should generally get care where they live.

Trajectories of Illness Across Time

How could health-care planning, financing, and policy identify and target the vulnerable population of people who have serious, progressive, chronic conditions that cause disability and suffering and will end in death? Specifically, for patients who are sick enough that death would not be surprising, would health-care services tailored to their particular needs improve their lives? If so, how are we to define the group and fit appropriate services to it? And, finally, does the process of tailoring services to patients' needs show us useful, informative divisions among those who are sick enough to die?

To answer these questions, it is helpful first to understand how to split the whole population into groups, according to what people in those groups generally need from the health-care system across time (Lynn 2001). The conventional divisions are by disease and setting of care. But these do not work well for a population that often has multiple diseases and needs multiple settings of care. Initially categorizing the entire population into the following three groups, as shown in the pie chart in figure 5, serves as a useful framework for organizing health care (Lunney, Lynn, and Hogan 2002; Lunney et al. 2003):

Healthy people and people with acute, time-limited conditions

People with stable or early chronic illness that is consistent with their usual social role and long life

People with serious, progressive, eventually fatal chronic illness (the "no surprise" population)

Priorities for generally healthy people and people with stable or mild chronic conditions are straightforward: to stay healthy, prevent disease, or restore good health. In these stages of life, people need mostly prevention and acute-care services (routine visits to health-care providers for prevention and health maintenance, and emergency medical services).

The third group, however—patients who live with serious chronic disease that will worsen and cause death—has much more complicated needs and priorities. People in this part of their lives still want to live as well as possible and usually for as long as possible. They and their families have many goals: relief from symptoms; help with family burdens; reasonable costs; ongoing good quality of life; a sense of being in control and maintaining dignity; and an opportunity to come to peace with spiritual issues and relationships. These goals coexist with those of preventing illness and prolonging life, even when pursuing such goals requires aggressive or invasive treatments. Holding all these goals simultaneously contrasts with the usual thinking that people near death need comfort and life closure, but not treatment. Instead of a "transition from cure to care," people living with fatal chronic illnesses have multiple complex goals and priorities that evolve over time.

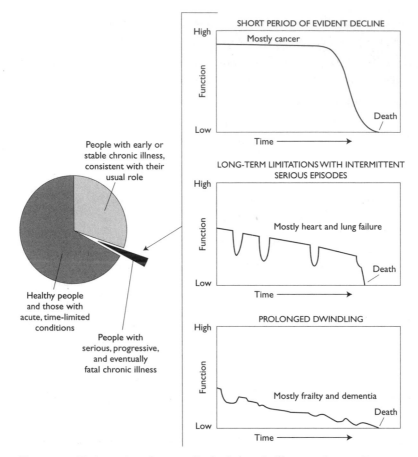

Figure 5. Trajectories of eventually fatal chronic illnesses. Source: Lynn and Adamson 2003.

Tailoring services to match the time course—or trajectory—of needs would be overwhelming if each disease and care setting required its own protocol. Conveniently, three patterns, illustrated in the three graphs in figure 5, appear to encompass most of the ways people traverse their time of living with chronic, progressive, eventually fatal conditions (Lunney, Lynn, and Hogan 2002).

SHORT PERIOD OF EVIDENT DECLINE — TYPICAL OF CANCER

Most patients with malignancies maintain comfort and functioning for a substantial period, even for several years following evidence of an eventually fatal condition. However, once the illness becomes overwhelming, their status usually declines quite rapidly in the weeks and days immediately preceding death (Morris et al. 1986). Because of this rather predictable course, such patients often have a period when their prognosis is reliably shorter than six months and thus they can qualify for hospice enrollment. Turning down "curative" treatment, as Medicare's hospice benefit requires, is largely symbolic; usually cure would never have been possible. However, most patients facing progressive cancer want to slow the cancer's progress and often have good functioning until very late in the course.

Many cancer patients become seriously disabled only with overwhelming disease, when the patient has only a few weeks to live. Having hospice services available to support patients and their caregivers during that concentrated period works reasonably well (Institute of Medicine 2001). About half of all cancer patients in the Medicare program now take advantage of hospice services (U.S. General Accounting Office 2000); these individuals represent about two-thirds of all the Medicare patients who use hospice (Gage and Dao 2000). Some cancers don't follow this trajectory because they regularly cause long-term disability rather than a short terminal decline (prostate cancer in elderly men, for example), and some other conditions (such as severe strokes, and some AIDS cases) follow this trajectory along with cancers.

CHRONIC ILLNESS WITH EXACERBATIONS AND SUDDEN DYING — TYPICAL OF ORGAN SYSTEM FAILURE

The second group of dying patients includes those with organ system failure, such as congestive heart failure (CHF), chronic obstructive pulmonary disease (COPD), cirrhosis, or kidney failure. They often live for a relatively long time following diagnosis and have long periods of staying in balance with the remaining organ system function. During those times, patients have few symptoms. But eventually some physiological stress overwhelms the body's reserves, leading to an exacerbation of serious symptoms.

Patients with organ system failure face an uncertain prognosis (Fox et al. 1999); most die suddenly from an unpredictable complication in the course of their chronic disease. The Study to Understand Prognoses and Preferences for Outcomes and Risks of Treatments (SUPPORT) found that most of these patients were stable and reasonably comfortable within a week of dying. The median heart failure patient still had a 50–50 chance to live six months, whether based on attending physicians' estimates or on a statistical model, on the day that turned out to be the patient's last full day alive (Lynn, Harrell, et al. 1997). In liver failure with cirrhosis, the median prognosis to survive six more months is approximately 4 in 10 within just two weeks before death (Roth et al. 2000). Death from emphysema is similarly difficult to predict, at least until the last few days (Claessens et al. 2000). The uncertainty of timing makes it appropriate to treat exacerbations as long as the patient is willing, even though treatment may fail and death follow. So the last phase of life for patients with this trajectory is much longer and indistinct, beginning at the point when the patient is first regularly limited by illness and continuing throughout recurrent exacerbations until death.

Close ongoing disease management has regularly proven to be effective in reducing exacerbations and improving survival span for patients with organ system failure (Rich et al. 1995; Bodenheimer et al. 2002). Many exacerbations arise from the patients' forgetting guidance about diet or medication, having insufficient funds to buy medications, or not understanding how to detect and treat early signs of an exacerbation. Programs that seek to prevent exacerbations and enhance quality of life generally emphasize self-care education, close symptom monitoring, around-the-clock on-call treatment of early symptoms, and consistent use of medications. Using quality-improvement methods, clinical teams have shown that adding advance care planning, mobilizing routine and urgent services to the home, and having deathbed care available at home yield further improvement in reducing exacerbations and costs and in tailoring services to patient and family preferences (Lynn, Schall, et al. 2000).

Because Medicare payments do not directly cover these services—though Medicare does cover hospitalization and emergency treatment—few people can get optimal care for serious organ system failure (Lynn, Wilkinson, and Etheredge 2001). Most patients following this trajectory are not homebound and so do not qualify for Medicare benefits for home care. In addition, these patients' prognoses are usually too uncertain for them to enroll in hospice programs. An individual physician or physician group could provide some of these services and be paid for office or home visits, but few physician practices have enough volume to support around-the-clock availability of a skilled person who knows the patient, has the patient's record, and could go to the home for timely evaluation and treatment. To justify the costs and ensure the skills, such a nursing service probably must enroll one hundred or more patients with similar organ system failure; thus implementation also requires limiting the number of provider organizations serving any one area. The United States does not have an established way to encourage concentrating services in a small number of providers in one area.

A LONG DWINDLING — TYPICAL OF FRAILTY AND DEMENTIA

Those who escape cancer and organ system failure are likely to die in late old age with generalized frailty of all body systems or neurological failure (such as Alzheimer's and other dementia). Alzheimer's dementia will likely affect fourteen million individuals in 2050 (Alzheimer's Association 2001). The final course for these patients is more appropriately characterized as a slow dwindling away, rather than the terminal course of many cancers or the intermittent exacerbations of organ system failures.

These patients are likely to lose the ability to take care of themselves long before death. As a result, they ordinarily require intensive personal care throughout their period of dependency, which imposes substantial burdens on both paid and volunteer (usually family) caregivers. These patients usually experience a slow worsening of self-care, with occasional episodes of more serious infections, injuries, or other illnesses. Some patients may get a substantial illness that takes life abruptly, especially when all concerned have decided not to pursue aggressive treatment to prolong life. Others continue to lose ground slowly and eventually die. Medical personnel do not generally classify someone as "dying" from dementia, Parkinson's disease, or just the multiple limitations of advanced old age. These patients tend to have uncertain prognoses and are therefore often not eligible for hospice under current coverage mechanisms (Hanrahan et al. 1999). Until the very last stages of their illness, they are not homebound and, consequently, do not qualify for Medicare benefits for home care. In the final stages of the disease, patients usually require very little skilled nursing, although they do require significant personal care, which Medicare or other health insurance does not cover.

Although these patients are difficult to fit into hospice or home-care nursing, an array of services has grown up to support the frail elderly and people with dementia. Care coordination services, Medicaid coverage of in-home and nursing-home personal care, Meals on Wheels, and other social service agencies fill some of the gap that would otherwise be left between conventional hospital and post-acute care on the one hand, and the real needs of these patients and their families on the other.

Frequency of Trajectories

Analyses of Medicare claims show that about one-fifth of those who die appear to have a disease likely to cause the first trajectory (a short decline in the last phase of life, mostly cancer), about one-fifth have illnesses associated with the second trajectory (sudden death in chronic organ system failure, mostly heart and lung), and about two-fifths have evidence

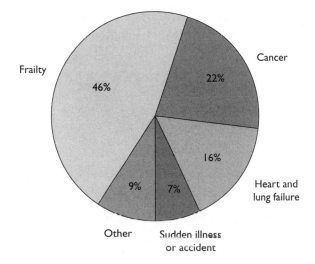

Figure 6.   Major medical conditions before death, for
Medicare beneficiaries. Source: Lunney, Lynn, and
Hogan 2002.

of a dwindling frailty course (figure 6). The rest are split between those
with very low expenses before death, indicating a likely sudden demise
(and also includes those getting services outside Medicare, mostly veter
ans) and a small group we have not yet learned to classify from claims
(Lunney, Lynn, and Hogan 2002). The groups' proportions are roughly
consistent with data from after-death interviews with families (Lunney et
al. 2003).

Some diagnoses may include patients who follow all three trajectories.
For instance, strokes can mark the onset of frailty and slow demise—but
sometimes multiple strokes and complications yield a course more like
organ system failure; or one devastating stroke kills the patient over a few
weeks, just as cancer can. Some types of cancer, such as prostate cancer
in the elderly, yield symptoms and time course that mimic frailty. AIDS
may evidence terminal cancer, intermittent infections and sudden dying,
or slow dementing illness.

Needs for care arise as disabilities and symptoms emerge; the service array should be based more on these needs than on diagnosis and prognosis. Categories designed to mesh with the likely time course of disability and suffering present a useful model for improving care. Hence, reform strategies based on these three major trajectories may be easier to envision, and more practical to accomplish, than strategies aimed at customizing a care system for every combination of illness(es) and site of care. Indeed, a quality-improvement project in Jönköping, Sweden, has adopted this model and is using it to learn how to serve the prototypical person in each of the three trajectories (QualityHealthCare.org 2003). Their claim is that if three paradigm patients—one with heart failure, one with colon cancer, and one with dementia (each named "Esther")—could all count on good care, then virtually everyone could count on good care. Thus, they are building a care system that delivers for all three.

The services that would match each trajectory have important common characteristics as well as differences (table 2). Clearly, every person coming to the end of his or her life needs to be confident of being comfortable, comforted, and in control of those elements of the experience that anyone can control. Those with rapidly declining clinical status in the first trajectory match the intensive but generally short-term services of hospice programs serving patients dying at home. Those with long-term chronic illnesses marked by periodic dramatic exacerbations need the self-care education, home-care support, medication management, and advance care planning that could constitute comprehensive disease management programs. Those with frailty and dementia and a long slow decline need respite for family caregivers, environmental accommodation for safety and ease of use, help with tasks of daily living, and eventually direct help with bathing and feeding. So care for those with serious, eventually fatal chronic illness could always include advance care planning and symptom management, while many other professional services would be customized to match the likely needs for each trajectory.

The proportion of people in each trajectory will shift with medical advances and lifestyle changes. As people reduce smoking and otherwise prevent lethal cancer, more people will live long enough to develop vas-

Table 2. *Priority care needs for the three illness trajectories*

For short period of evident decline (mostly cancer)
- Adapting services to rapid changes in the patient
- Controlling symptoms
- Providing support for families: training, respite, and counseling through bereavement
- Ensuring continuity of the clinical team
- Life closure and completion

For chronic illness with intermittent exacerbations and sudden dying (mostly organ system failure)
- Preventing exacerbations and providing early treatment
- Planning for urgent situations
- Making decisions about the benefits of low-yield treatments
- Mobilizing services to the home
- Preparing families for sudden death
- Life closure and completion

For slow dwindling (mostly frailty and dementia)
- Fostering caregiver endurance, loyalty, and reliability
- Providing long-term personal care services and supervision
- Helping family caregivers to find meaning and avoid severe burdens
- Avoiding undesired prolongation of life
- Keeping skin intact
- Finding pleasurable moments to enjoy
- Life closure and completion

cular and heart disease. To the extent that prevention (through diet, medications, and exercise) is effective for heart disease, more people will live long enough to encounter dementia and frailty. Dying from cancer tends to peak around seventy years of age, and heart and lung disease about a decade later. Most people who survive past eighty-five eventually need daily care and accumulate evidence of multisystem lack of reserves. Thus, to the extent that prevention and early treatment are successful, more Americans are likely to live their last years with frailty and dementia.

Recent reports suggest a modest diminution of serious disability in old age (Crimmins, Saito, and Reynolds 1997; Manton, Corder, and Stallard 1997; Manton and Gu 2001), but this cannot mean major changes in the overall care needs of the elderly. Better geriatric care might be able to provide rehabilitation and environmental changes that enable people to care for themselves for longer periods. In addition, the disabilities of arthritis, hearing and vision deficits, and dentition problems may be amenable to prevention and amelioration. However, since general frailty is the most common course to death in advanced old age, patients regularly experience years of serious disability before dying.

Anticipating Challenges

Advance care planning is the way to ensure that the patient and family get to shape many details of the care plan, if they want to do so (Teno and Lynn 1996). The person who wants to die without an attempt at resuscitation needs to have the opportunity to say so. Some patients want to control who is in the room—both to include and to exclude. Having the right medications to treat serious symptoms may require storing them at the home and ensuring that someone has the skills to give them when needed. Again, advance care planning can allow choices over many things, both the medical treatment issues and the small details of importance to the patient.

The health-care system has certain routine responses to serious complications—resuscitation for circulatory cessation, transfusion for bleeding, or antibiotics for pneumonia, for example. Most of these are, quite reasonably, aimed at restoring or preserving health. But these can be difficult or burdensome interventions, and seriously ill persons nearing the end of life often do not want and will not benefit from them. Avoiding them requires explicit planning in advance.

Thus, advance care planning is mainly thinking ahead: considering the likely course and the unlikely, but potentially important, complications; and making plans for how to live as well as one can through what is coming. It is not merely a statement as to who should make decisions when the patient cannot, nor is it just a decision about resuscitation or hospitalization, though those are important. Fundamentally, advance care planning requires thinking about the future and putting in place the specific arrangements that will improve the likelihood that the patient and family will live out the last phase of life in the way that is meaningful to them. Obviously, advance care planning is an essential part of good care for serious chronic illness.

Creating and Naming a Category

Tailoring services to match the needs of the last phase of life requires defining that phase in useful ways. Certain considerations shape the care system for all three trajectories:

Living well with serious chronic illnesses until death is a worthy goal—alongside prevention and cure of illnesses, and delay of disability and death.

Serious chronic illnesses require continuity and comprehensiveness of care, with flexibility to adjust to the resources and preferences of patients and their families as well as their varying health-care needs.

Because the timing of death remains quite unpredictable until very late in the course of serious chronic illnesses, diagnosis and severity—not prognosis—must trigger special arrangements for care near the end of life.

Efficient and reliable care systems might differentiate on the basis of the service needs of the three trajectories by disability and symptoms over time, rather than by location of care or by diagnosis.

The major causes of death are all progressive, degenerative illnesses that leave people in fragile health for a long period of time before dying.

Any major success in treating or preventing any of the major medical conditions of the end of life will only delay, not circumvent,
the need for end-of-life care, since most elderly people have multiple competing causes of death. Even if one cause of death entirely vanished, another would take its place after a relatively
short delay.

This shift toward serious chronic disease as the way that Americans come
to the end of life has not been sudden. So why has it taken so long to adapt
our social models and services to fit the needs of patients who will be very
sick for a long time? Three factors have contributed to our failure to change:

First, many Americans do not understand what happens to people as
they approach the end of life. This misunderstanding derives in
part from media stereotypes of death and dying and a matching
lack of personal experience with old age, serious illness, and
dying.

Second, our system of financing health care developed two generations ago, in the 1950s and 1960s, when the top priorities were
relieving the barriers to diagnostic and surgical procedures. The
drive to stave off illness indefinitely and ensure access to medical
miracles left little consideration of programs to serve people living with eventually fatal chronic illnesses.

Third, the structure of the Medicare hospice benefit, which offers
an alternative to conventional care but is available only when
death within six months is virtually certain, reinforces the image
that people will die "on time." Doctors classify only certain types
of patients as "dying" and as being eligible for hospice services.
But many patients who die without having enrolled in hospice
would benefit from hospicelike services, if such services were
available for up to several years of tenuous survival before death.

While people who are generally healthy might also benefit from all-
inclusive care over time, comprehensiveness and continuity are lower

priorities because healthy people are able to seek diagnosis and treatment using their own ability to follow through, make judgments, pursue opportunities, and marshal resources. In contrast, many patients and families who need help to live with a serious chronic condition are not nearly as capable of patching together workable care and treatment arrangements. People who are sick enough to die should not have to customize their own care system; the care system should make it almost automatic to get the services that enable people to live well through a period of serious disability before death. That goal is challenging but not out of reach. The complexity of these patients' goals, the uncertainty of their life span, and the difficulties they face in advocating for their own well-being mean that the community and its professionals should shape a care system that fits the needs of people going through this phase of life, rather than make these needs fit the current hospital-centered arrangement.

There is no simple label for this category yet. Some favor the term "serious and complex condition" (Institute of Medicine 1999a). I prefer (and often use) "eventually fatal chronic illness" (Myers and Lynn 2002). Either term certainly takes in far more than patients who have a "terminal illness" in the sense that their dying is predictable and close. Instead, the category includes those who have serious and progressive chronic conditions that will generally keep them in substantially compromised health for all of the rest of their lives.

Such tailored care for the last phase of life cannot address only "comfort care," nor can it be available only to people who have a prognosis of dying quickly. Virtually every person with chronic lung failure (for example, emphysema) would be well advised to make plans about whether or not to use ventilator support for the next exacerbation of symptoms, even though much time could pass before the issue arises (Lynn, Schuster, and Kabcenell 2000; Lynn and Goldstein 2003). Likewise, many of these patients would fare better if they had the wrap-around support services now routinely provided only in hospice, such as prescription drug coverage, spiritual counseling, continuity, bereavement support, symptom prevention and relief, home health aides, and family support (National Hospice and Palliative Care Organization and Center to Advance Palliative Care 2001).

More Patients, Fewer Caregivers

The daunting numbers of people with serious disability and fatal chronic illness and the shortage of family and paid caregivers should make greater availability of skilled caregivers a priority over the coming decade. Since large numbers of disabled elderly in 2030 will first experience the dysfunctions of care when they serve as family caregivers, they might then be motivated to political action to rebuild the care system to be more reliable. Compared to their parents, baby boomers tend to be more aware of health issues (Kennedy 1998) and far more aggressive in demanding the services that meet needs (Bartlett 1999). The aging of this group presents not only daunting challenges but also powerful leverage for activism. As the Institute for the Future (2000) points out, "Baby Boomers have transformed many institutions and aspects of society along their life cycle—including the workplace, financial institutions, and government. As Baby Boomers interact with the health-care system, their expectations and preferences will also transform these institutions as the health-care industry adapts to accommodate Baby Boomers' demands and numbers." Certainly the very sick living out the end of their lives have little direct political force. But their family members might have more, and the baby boomer generation has every reason to seek better solutions, since it will be the next to use them.

Working Out Patterns of Costs

What we know about the costs and use of health services near the end of life presents an interesting picture. The proportion of Medicare costs spent on the last year of life, or the last month, has stayed nearly constant for two decades. Other than for chronic renal failure, average costs for the last year decline sharply with age but are quite similar across all major diagnoses. End-stage renal failure has always been a costly way to live and to die, with average Medicare costs over $50,000 for all years, including the year of death (Hogan et al. 2000). All other major causes of death for people ages sixty-five to seventy-five cost about $26,000 (in 1997 dollars) in their last year. The fact that the major ways to die converge on a small range of average costs is quite curious. Perhaps the care system does not commonly implement more services than providers and caregivers consider decent and appropriate. It is an intriguing possibility that awaits more research.

Whereas being sick enough to die (and being covered by Medicare) trumps most of the biases that relate to wealth, race, income, and gender (Shugarman et al. 2004), variations in patients' age and in geography continue to correlate with major differences in costs. The decline in hospitalization and physician services as patients age may reflect fewer opportunities to affect frailty and dementia. Of course, the decline may also reflect age bias in offering care or older patients' and families' increasing preference for comfort. The differences in use by similar patients in different parts of the country might arise from differences in the availability of services, a possibility that has substantial support in the literature (Last Acts 2002; Dartmouth Atlas of Health Care 1999).

Perhaps the very different patterns between areas also reflect real differences in what communities feel is essential to good care and in how different parts of the care system are set to respond (Dartmouth Atlas of Health Care 1999). In Oregon, for instance, providers are proud of keeping very sick people well supported at home. Hospice is readily available, around the clock, almost everywhere. Adult foster care homes aim to keep their residents in place. Patients, their families, and care teams see going into the hospital with an incurable condition as a loss. In New York, the same act of treating sick people where they live might lead to allegations of mistreatment by the nursing facility or home-care team. Hospice care at home is not common. In my experience, New Yorkers often feel that hospitals are best for treating sick people and that nursing homes and other settings for geriatric care are generally more risky settings for care. Thus, the variations in practice in different areas might arise from variations in the supply of services and possibilities for income, or they might depend on communities' expectations and capabilities. Most likely, factors such as these are mutually supportive and together create barriers to change. Nevertheless, the fact that geography has a greater effect on costs than diagnosis or wealth should help illuminate possibilities for change: sometimes to address inadequate services, often to challenge costly approaches on the basis of efficiency.

Summary of Ideas to Shape Reform

We are all still learning how to respond to our new way of living at the end of life. The care system shaped in the decades after World War II aimed to provide surgeries and other dramatic interventions to most of the population, and it largely succeeds. Indeed, its success is part of what led to the burgeoning numbers of patients and families who face serious chronic disease in old age.

Our very language of care no longer fits the population and its needs. Policy makers ordinarily operate without the data they need to establish goals and priorities in this area or even to assess the effects of changes. Federal health agencies working amid competing priorities have little time for innovations in end-of-life care; indeed, our leaders of medicine and public health do not yet fully realize that health care concentrates more and more on supporting people with fatal chronic illness. Many patients and families still do not know what to ask of their health-care providers.

Even those seeking reform in this area are split among advocacy groups on aging, disability, hospice, nursing homes, rehabilitation, and individual diseases. Most services in the current health-care system are not tailored to meet the needs of individuals with serious, eventually fatal chronic illness. The gaps in our care system place these vulnerable patients at risk for unrelieved pain, indignity, and powerlessness and also burden and impoverish their families. Yet few organizations take up the cause.

Some better ideas have been emerging to remedy these deficiencies, including some important revisions of conventional wisdom. The changes in clinical, institutional, and financing policy this chapter has presented could be the foundations for a reliable care system that serves people living with serious chronic disease in the last phase of life.

We will see data differently if we bear in mind that people get to live bounded lives, not to live on indefinitely. Success in prevention, public health, and health care have led to putting most of the burden of illness on the last few years of life, which is a laudable accomplishment that creates new challenges.

The claim that people generally move from wanting to live and receive medical care to accepting death and wanting hospice care is a widespread but misleading social construction of reality. The more accurate and useful claim is that most patients facing serious chronic illnesses have decreasing opportunities to delay progression of their illnesses and increasing needs to live well despite those illnesses.

Since most people in this last phase of life have multiple health problems, diagnoses and cause of death are more complex but less relevant than when people generally had one serious problem at a time.

Since most people will need multiple settings for care (home, hospital, nursing home), integration and linkages among these settings are essential to quality care. Measuring quality requires focusing on a population in need (like those living with advanced heart failure) rather than only a setting of care (such as nursing homes).

Services tailored to the end of life can target people who are seriously ill or disabled, with a generally worsening condition (or conditions) that will cause death. This last part of most lives requires long-term services, complex balancing of priorities, and increasing support for personal care.

Clinicians can identify the target population with the "no surprise" question: would it be no surprise if this sick person died within the coming year (or the coming few months)? Asking for a reliable prognosis of less than six months, as the Medicare hospice benefit requires, identifies only a small proportion of the population and generally does so long after these individuals have started to suffer from eventually fatal chronic illnesses.

Trajectories of disease or disability usefully divide the population with eventually fatal chronic illness into three groups:

- Short period of evident decline, typical of cancers
- Long-term limitations with intermittent serious episodes (and sudden dying), typical of organ system failures
- Prolonged dwindling, typical of dementia, disabling strokes, and frailty of old age

Advance care planning is useful not only for allowing care decisions to proceed when the patient is incompetent but also for avoiding specific and otherwise automatic responses of the health-care system to illness and complications, and for putting in place the concrete services that ensure implementation of preferred options.

The number of persons living with eventually fatal chronic illnesses will increase dramatically over the coming quarter century. The paucity of family and paid caregivers is already evident and likely to worsen. The obvious crisis of caregiving generates substantial challenges and opportunities for creative steps toward reliable and sustainable care arrangements.

Quality Comes Home
Donald M. Berwick

My father was a retired physician in rural Connecticut. For 42 years, he provided care as a general practitioner in the tiny town in which I grew up. Then he retired and found himself no longer giving care but receiving it. I do not know what he thought of health care reform. By the time the national issue became popular, my father was mentally unable to comprehend the debate. . . .

He was the guy who got up in the middle of the night because Jimmy had a high fever, or Mr. Bernstein had a heart attack, or an awful car accident occurred at the drawbridge. . . . When I attended my 30th high school reunion in 1994, I was still Dr. Berwick's boy. People could not wait to remind me of the time my father delivered their baby or themselves, or sewed a wound, or answered a tough question. They called him a great doctor. He was always there, they said. You could count on him.

My father retired in 1984 and not long afterward began developing symptoms of Parkinson disease and mild dementia from small, multiple strokes. He remained alert but became progressively weaker until he fell at home and broke his hip in June of 1994. . . .

One of my brothers, who lives an hour from our father's home, rushed to the local hospital to meet him in the emergency department. He was told—in error—that our father was not there. Panicked telephone calls followed as my brother searched anxiously for our father's whereabouts until, finally, someone told him that our father was there, after all, and was about to be wheeled into the operating room.

After surgery, my father lay sedated on a special mattress containing sections that alternately inflated and deflated. Within a week, he had a deep pressure ulcer on his right heel. It was painful and interrupted his early ambulation therapy. He became restricted to a wheelchair for most of the day and gradually refused to walk at all. Unable to return home, my father needed to go to a rehabilitation facility. . . .

I visited him there on the morning after his admission. He was lying stuporous in the bed, on his back, with his ulcerated heel pressing into the sheets. His mouth was hanging open, and his eyes were rolled back into his head. I asked the nurse for an explanation. "We sedated him," she said. "He was combative. He hit a staff member." For 10 years, my father had had severe Parkinson disease, and for most of that time he had been unable to voluntarily extend his own arm, much less throw a roundhouse punch. My father had undoubtedly been angry, yes. But a punch . . . no. I demanded that the sedation be stopped.

Not that it mattered much. For reasons that never became clear, the medication he took for Parkinson disease, meticulously adjusted for 2 years by his physician at home, was summarily stopped when he was admitted to the rehabilitation facility. This resulted in a 2-week siege of spasm and much decreased mobility. Not that that mattered much, either. By then, the pressure sore on his right heel had opened again, causing pain that prevented him from walking or even spending much time in a wheelchair.

Not that it mattered, because when my brothers and I asked that our father be placed in a wheelchair whenever possible, the nurses on the weekend shift told us that no wheelchairs could be found. They asked that we bring in his rickety old wheelchair from home. They eventually did find a wheelchair, but it was missing the footrest plate that would have protected his injured heel from bruising.

My father spent 6 weeks in the rehabilitation facility and then gave up, as did the staff. He returned home to a hospital bed and around-the-clock housekeeper coverage. Two weeks after he returned home—almost entirely bedridden and almost certainly never to walk again—a wheelchair finally came: the latest model, with postural supports, custom back rests, and hand controls he could never use. It was beautiful. The price: $6000. It sat proudly and nearly totally unused in the corner of his bedroom. . . .

My father did not care. He was in bed with a pressure sore, staring at a wheelchair he did not need and living with the undeserved memory of insult, delay, and medically induced coma.

If we cannot work together on improvements that matter to those who call on us for help, then we have no cause to take pride in our restructuring, our mergers, our integrated systems, or our report cards. I propose that we take aim where it matters. Pressure sores are the enemy. Stop them. Errors in drug use are the enemy. Stop them. Fragmentation is the enemy. It creates waste, cost, and disrespect. Stop it. It was my father this time, but next time it will be your father, and then you, and then your child. I have heard it said by cynics that the quality of medical care would be far better and the hazards far less if physicians, like pilots, were passengers in their own airplanes. We are.

Adapted with permission from Berwick DM. 1996. Quality comes home. *Ann Intern Med.* 125:839–843.

3

GOOD CARE FOR SOME
PEOPLE, SOMETIMES

Reformers have already tried out some important innovations, including projects showing that patients with serious chronic illness regularly benefit from continuity and coordinated care in which each provider in each setting knows the patient's diagnosis, treatment plan, and preferences. These innovations and reforms are useful not only for what they have achieved for small numbers of people or short periods of time but also for what they can teach about organizing reliable, high-quality care (National Coalition for Health Care and Institute for Healthcare Improvement 2000; Romer et al. 2002; Lynn, Schuster, and Kabcenell 2000). Professional education, health-care provider regulation and certification, and collaborative quality-improvement efforts are making strides toward practical reforms (End of Life/Palliative Education Resource Center 2001; Education for Physicians on End-of-Life Care Project 2000; End-of-Life Nursing Education Consortium 2000; Joint Commission on Accreditation of Healthcare Organizations 2001; Lynn, Schall, et al. 2000; Du Pen et al. 1999). Some programs that began as demonstration models have proven their merit and have become part of routine care: for example, hospice and the Program of All-Inclusive Care for the Elderly (PACE).

Optimal management of the chronically ill or frail elderly requires comprehensive multidimensional assessment of medical, functional, and psychosocial needs; arrangement of community services; coordination across providers; intensive health education and support for lifestyle modification; and methodical tracking of patients' progress between of-

66

fice visits (Chen et al. 2000). A variety of approaches have made some real gains toward ensuring these services. This chapter reviews important insights from these instructive innovations.

Hospice

America's version of hospice services arose largely as a reaction to the inadequate care of the "dying" in the 1970s and early 1980s. Rather than let doctors and hospitals dominate care for these patients, hospice relied on community-based, volunteer, and family-centered care. At a time when cancer patients' pain was rarely treated adequately, hospice offered aggressive, around-the-clock pain management in the form of adequate doses of opioids and comfort measures for other symptoms. And at a time when the suffering brought by cancer, radiation, and chemotherapy made many patients wish for early death, hospice offered patients and families the opportunity to live on the patients' own terms. The results of this strategy were dramatic, with testimonials abounding as to its merits. When Medicare began to pay for hospice services in 1983 (42 CFR Part 418), the legislation clearly structured hospice as an alternative to conventional care. For example, the law required explicit and careful consent from patients, acknowledging that they were giving up "curative" treatment. Patients who transferred to hospice, and those who cared for them, viewed the transfer as a renunciation of the chance for cure and a clear shift toward accepting death.

In the twenty years since the Medicare hospice benefit was enacted, hospice has become a routine part of health care, at least for adults with terminal cancer. In 2002, about 25 percent of Americans who died used hospice (885,000 hospice users) for a median of twenty-six days (and a mean of fifty-one days) (National Hospice and Palliative Care Organization 2003a). Hospice care often enables people to die at home, the place most Americans say they would prefer to die (Gallup Organization 1996; Fried et al. 1999; Pritchard et al. 1998; Groth-Juncker and Mc-Cusker 1983). The Medicare hospice benefit requires an interdisciplinary team including at least a physician, a nurse, and a social worker to work with patients and families to articulate a care plan. While the hospice model of care has had only a little rigorous or generalizable evaluation, the public perception of hospice is strongly favorable.

Nevertheless, few people are aware of hospice or understand its benefits. Nearly 80 percent of Americans do not think of hospice as a choice for end-of-life care. Approximately 75 percent do not know that hospice care can be provided at home. More than 90 percent do not know that hospice provides pain relief for the terminally ill, or that Medicare pays for hospice (National Hospice and Palliative Care Organization 2003b). People who are aware of hospice usually think of its services as being a blessing in a desperate situation.

Hospice programs generally receive an all-inclusive per diem rate, about $100 per day for routine home care (National Hospice and Palliative Care Organization 2003b) and more for in-patient or extensive care. At least 80 percent of days must be at the basic home-care rate. Services usually include assessment and treatment by a nurse and physician, as well as home health care, social work, spiritual and bereavement counseling, pharmacy and durable medical equipment, and other therapies as appropriate. While Medicare officially classifies hospice as a fee-for-service benefit (paying a fee for a day of service), the programs operate with many characteristics of managed care—paying for services from a pool collected from per diem payments and controlling admissions and expenses to keep an operating margin in the pool of funds.

Under Medicare, hospice programs are effectively available to Medicare beneficiaries in all parts of the country (Hogan 2001). Hospice covers prescription medications that are related to the terminal illness (with a small co-pay), which creates inducements for patients to enroll and necessitates that hospices take steps to control medication expenditures in order to remain solvent. Indeed, many hospice programs will not pay for certain costly or invasive treatments, a position that may be rooted in hospice's philosophy of care but is certainly buttressed by the need to devise a workable business plan.

As it enters its third decade of service in the United States, hospice is stabilizing after several years of serious confrontation with fraud investigations, which originated from the Medicare requirement that patients have a prognosis of less than six months. Several years ago, the Office of the Inspector General (OIG) of the U.S. Department of Health and Human Services (1997) investigated several situations in which many patients in a program outlived their six-month prognosis. The OIG alleged that the hospice should have predicted long stays on the day of admission (and therefore should not have enrolled the patients). As a result of this investigation, some hospices and physicians have become more reluctant to risk enrolling patients whose prognoses are unclear.

Despite its many merits, the current hospice Medicare benefit puts the program out of reach for most of the time that patients are seriously ill with eventually fatal illnesses, in part because their prognoses are uncertain. In 2001, 54 percent of hospice deaths were cancer patients, with the remainder of hospice deaths largely distributed among five disease categories: heart disease (10 percent), dementia (7 percent), lung disease (6 percent), kidney disease (3 percent), and liver failure (2 percent) (National Hospice and Palliative Care Organization 2003b). Because patients in the second and third trajectories toward death (organ system failure, frailty and dementia, as discussed in chapter 2) often have virtually no period when it can be determined that they are very likely to die within six months, physicians do not think to refer them to hospice care. Indeed, the patients and their families are not likely to have a period when they see themselves as being appropriate for hospice care. Thus, although hospice is a valued model for the patients it serves, it cannot serve many individuals on many of the days when they could benefit from hospice's comprehensive, home-based services.

Support for the claim that hospice improves care consists mainly of anecdotal reports. One survey of family survivors attests to the merits of hospice services for nursing-home residents (Baer and Hanson 2000). Teno and colleagues (2004) reported that family members, about one year after the patient's death, remembered the time near death as much better supported when using hospice care at home than in all other settings. While some early and methodologically limited studies indicated that hospice use might save money (Mor and Kidder 1985; National Hospice Organization 1995), a recent study indicates that hospice tends to be cost-neutral for most cancer patients and cost-adding for most noncancer patients (Campbell et al. 2004). Understanding the interactions of various service strategies for end-of-life care (including nursing facility, home care, hospital, and hospice) and defining the structures that optimally balance costs and outcomes would require focused studies that have not yet been undertaken.

Nevertheless, hospice experience to date shows that the public can accept—and even welcome—a program of care that focuses upon dying people and tries to support patients and families in the home. Hospice repeatedly demonstrates that paid and unpaid caregivers can be recruited and that they find such work to be rewarding. Many programs now recruit teenagers and older adults to assist their neighbors (National Coalition for Health Care and Institute for Healthcare Improvement 2000). Furthermore, the financial arrangements used in Medicare hospice may provide a model for structuring a new benefit for comprehensive home-care services to all people with serious, eventually fatal chronic illness (see trajectories of achievable excellence in chapter 5).

Palliative Care at Home

Several innovative programs have developed strategies to improve links between home health care, disease management programs, and hospice and palliative care (National Coalition for Health Care and Institute for Healthcare Improvement 2002). At a Kaiser Permanente facility in southern California, for example, the hospice and palliative-care team worked with staff members from a disease management program to improve end-of-life care (Brumley, Enguidanos, and Cherin 2003). The Kaiser Bellflower program aimed to improve families' satisfaction, increase the number of patients referred for hospice care, reduce the need for 911 calls and emergency room admissions, and identify dying patients earlier in the course of their illness. The program developed a checklist to guide hospice staff during home visits to patients with advanced heart and lung failure. It also worked on outreach to all subspecialty physicians in Kaiser medical centers and encouraged physicians to refer seriously ill patients to hospice while patients were in stable, outpatient settings, rather than waiting for an emergency situation. Finally, the program designated liaison nurses to provide one-on-one training and information to physicians throughout the system. Over an eight-month period, emergency transport calls and unplanned hospitalizations went from four per hundred patients to fewer than two per hundred (National Coalition for Health Care and Institute for Healthcare Improvement 2002).

Palliative Care in Hospitals

Nearly 70 percent of all deaths in New York City occur in hospitals, and 63 percent of these deaths are among patients age sixty-five or older. Yet very few receive comprehensive palliative care (Zuckerman and Mackinnon 1998). In response to this statistic, the United Hospital Fund implemented its Hospital Palliative Care Initiative to share information about end-of-life care in hospitals. In addition, New York's Mount Sinai School of Medicine launched a palliative-care program in 1997 to give patients access to palliative-care services and to educate new physicians, house staff, fellows, and medical students (National Coalition for Health Care and Institute for Healthcare Improvement 2000). That model gave Mount Sinai the experience to lead the Center to Advance Palliative Care (CAPC), which helps hospitals nationwide to establish palliative-care services (Center to Advance Palliative Care 2000b).

A decade ago, almost no hospitals had programs directed at palliative care. Now, nearly one-fifth of community hospitals and one-fourth of teaching hospitals have some sort of program in place, and many more are being planned (Center to Advance Palliative Care 2000a). In fact, in 2002 the American Hospital Association reported a 20 percent increase in the number of hospital-based palliative-care programs over the previous year (Center to Advance Palliative Care 2003). These programs are providing substantial consultation services for hospitalized patients, and they are being supported by billings, grants, and subsidization by the hospital (Milbank Memorial Fund and Robert Wood Johnson Foundation 2000). Some programs have generated special units whose staff members receive special training and orientation, while others take care of people throughout the hospital, wherever they happen to be. Certain programs have special expertise in symptom control (especially pain from cancer), others in decision making and family counseling (especially for geriatric patients), and a few in special services for ventilator withdrawal (Coyle 1997; Campbell and Frank 1997).

Because various models of palliative care match the needs of varying situations, many models are in place. Services that a particular hospital should develop must be a function of several variables including resource potential, population needs, and availability of staff trained in palliative care (Center to Advance Palliative Care 2000b). No specific funding supports these programs yet. Physicians' billings for consultations and procedures have been the backbone of most budgets, along with philanthropic funds. In many hospital settings, the shortened length of stay and reduced use of redundant, unnecessary, or ineffective tests and pharmaceuticals have been enough to make palliative care a good investment for the hospital (Center to Advance Palliative Care 2000a; Smith et al. 2003). Many facilities clearly see the value of palliative-care expertise, which serves perceived needs in a way that was not otherwise possible (National Hospice and Palliative Care Organization and Center to Advance Palliative Care 2001).

Case Study
Project Safe Conduct (Circle of Life award winner)

Begun as a demonstration project in palliative care, Project Safe Conduct is a collaborative venture between Hospice of the Western Reserve, a large community-based hospice, and Ireland Cancer Center, a National Cancer Institute comprehensive cancer center at University Hospitals of Cleveland. The innovation of this venture lies in having an external palliative-care team from a hospice housed within a cancer center and integrated into its system of care.

The interdisciplinary team includes a nurse with advanced training, a social worker, and a spiritual-care counselor. It works with the oncology team at the Ireland Cancer Center and has access to pain specialists and psychologists for consultation. The team introduced a pain-care pathway and guidelines for pain management, as well as a flow sheet for tracking pain assessment and management. To increase continuity of care, the program has a team member present at every clinic appointment for each patient and makes a patient consultation hotline available during weekday business hours.

The Safe Conduct team advocates for patients regarding their care, with a particular focus on helping them recognize moments that might be key decision points. In order to ensure that patients get the most appropriate care at the right time, the team holds family conferences early in the disease trajectory. Communication is part of every phase of care; team members work with patients and families to make sure that they understand the implications of test results and that the physician understands their concerns.

After the demonstration project's funding ended, Ireland Cancer Center integrated the team into standard practice.

To obtain further information, visit www.irelandcancercenter.org/ PatientCareTeamsICC-thoracic-safeConductTeam.htm.

Innovations in End-of-Life Care. 2002. Executive summary of 2002 Circle of Life award winner. June. Adapted with permission from *Innovations in End-of-Life Care* online magazine, Education Development Center, Inc.

PACE: All-Inclusive Care

The Program of All-Inclusive Care of the Elderly extends its comprehensive housing, personal, and health-care services to persons eligible for nursing-home care, mostly under a dual capitation from Medicare and Medicaid (capitation involves a uniform per capita payment, regardless of treatment individual patients require; a few patients pay Medicaid's part on their own). Because they must be disabled and nursing-home eligible, PACE patients are almost always living with an eventually fatal chronic condition. PACE is not seen as an end-of-life service, and there are no prognostic requirements for enrollment. But PACE programs cannot discharge enrollees except for a few unusual reasons, so most patients die while in the program and are substantially disabled throughout. PACE is small but illuminating as a program targeted at the last years of life, mostly to people in a frailty trajectory.

PACE programs provide the following services (National PACE Association 2003):

Adult day care with therapists (physical, occupational, and recreational) and nursing care

Meals and nutritional counseling

Social work and personal care

Comprehensive primary medical care provided by a PACE physician

Services of medical specialists, including audiology, dentistry, optometry, podiatry, and speech therapy

Home health care and personal care

All necessary prescription drugs

Social services

Respite care

Hospital and nursing-home care when necessary

Using interdisciplinary teams, the PACE program is responsible for all services that Medicare or Medicaid would have provided. PACE programs pool all payments from Medicare, Medicaid, and private sources to create a single fund to pay for all covered and supplementary services, giving programs substantial flexibility in services provided. PACE programs can use their funds to support day care, housing adaptations, disposable supplies, and other elements that are not part of the standard "package" of covered services.

In 2002, twenty-eight PACE sites and ten pre-PACE (in development) sites served more than ten thousand patients around the country (National PACE Association 2002). The majority of these patients are quite old and very frail. The profile of a typical PACE participant is like that of the average nursing-home resident: she is eighty years old, has about eight chronic medical conditions, and needs help with three activities of daily living (such as mobility, dressing, and toileting). Among PACE participants, 49 percent have been diagnosed with dementia (National PACE Association 2000). In 2001, PACE received $1.3 million in federal funding for expansion efforts.

Formal evaluation of PACE is under way, and initial reports show good rates of satisfaction with the services and uncertain effects upon costs of care (White, Abel, and Kidder 2000). A 1997 study of Medicare's expenditures for a comparably elderly and frail population found that PACE yields Medicare a 12 percent savings (Gruenberg and Kaganova 1997). In 1998, the median Medicare capitation rate for PACE was $1,226 per enrollee per month, with a range of $877 to $1,775, depending on locale (Catholic Health Association 2003). The Medicaid contribution varies much more, being set by each state. The PACE sites are quite varied in their services, patients enrolled, and setting (Temkin-Greener and Mukamel 2002).

PACE programs emphasize socialization, recreation, rehabilitation to maintain function, and secondary prevention. The success of PACE programs in meeting the needs of frail elders offers lessons in how to care for people facing death as a result of dementia or frailty. The PACE program has demonstrated the effectiveness of creating a flexible program that is tailored to the needs of individual patients and families.

While other programs struggle to provide continuity and comprehensive care, PACE has learned to rely on all of its staff members to monitor participants' health and to watch for signs that a person may be failing. For instance, drivers who pick up patients to attend PACE centers watch for changes in patients' mobility and report these to health-care staff.

PACE has been slow to grow to serve more people, despite substantial support from philanthropies and the federal government. Patients sometimes resist referral, often fearing loss of their usual doctor and sometimes resisting use of the adult day-care center. States have been slow to set Medicaid rates, in part because PACE's focus on out-of-hospital care can effectively shift costs from Medicare-covered hospitalization to Medicaid-covered supportive care. Mostly, though, slow growth probably reflects resistance to change, even with evidence of improved care. Early evaluations of the model have shown that it reduces the use of hospitals and nursing homes. Yet PACE has proven difficult to implement, recruitment has been slow, and its net effects on total health-care costs and on patients' functional ability and health status are not yet clear (Boult et al. 2000).

Other interventions aiming to provide more comprehensive management of chronic illness patients have included interdisciplinary home care, disease management, ACE units (hospital-based acute care for elders), geriatric evaluation and management, and case management.

The Chronic-Care Model

Wagner and his colleagues have developed a model of optimal chronic care, for use as a universally applicable guide to fundamental reforms that aim to improve outcomes for individuals living with chronic illness (Bodenheimer, Wagner, and Grumbach 2002a; Bodenheimer, Wagner, and Grumbach 2002b; Robert Wood Johnson Foundation 2000). Implementing it requires managing and organizing the care system, most often through a staff-model managed-care plan like Group Health of Puget

Sound, where the model originated. Essentially the same model guides revisions at a number of integrated delivery systems that include at least hospital, office practice, and home care.

The model focuses on the collaboration between each knowledgeable and motivated patient and his or her care team in the comprehensive, ongoing management of the patient's chronic illness(es). The care system is responsible for developing registries of patients and using them to ensure timely preventive and maintenance services. Since patients are central to managing their own conditions, the model directs attention to ensuring that patients are capable of self-care (Robert Wood Johnson Foundation 2000; Bodenheimer et al. 2002). In addition, the implementation of the model depends on effective information technology.

The chronic-care model has gathered enough support to spur foundations and clinical sites to become engaged in related implementation and evaluation activities (such as Improving Chronic Illness Care and Partnership for Solutions). At least some applications of this model appear to be effective in improving patient experience and system efficiency (Davis, Wagner, and Groves 2000; Wagner et al. 1999; Coleman et al. 1999). But the model has primarily been applied in managed-care settings that do not have many elderly patients, and younger patients are not often in the advanced stages of illness. Thus, the merits of the model have not been directly addressed with the sickest patients, and the model does not highlight issues of special relevance to people near death, such as advance care planning, mobilizing services to the home, family support, or symptom control. Even so, the Medicare reform legislation in 2003 provided for improved projects around this model and for managed-care plans focused upon special-needs populations (Medicare Prescription Drug, Improvement, and Modernization Act 2003). Additionally, the way in which the chronic-care model directs investments in information systems, registries, and self-management support has been an important force for reform of the usual doctor's office, with its paper records and inability to track preventive services or to provide training for self-care.

Coordinating and Managing Care

Patients with serious chronic illness often see many specialists and other health-care professionals in a range of settings. Coordination of care for these patients among providers and across provider sites is important to avoid complications (such as monitoring drug interactions or transfer of patient-care plan across settings), but health-care systems rarely provide this service. The fragmentation and disorganization of the fee-for-service health-care system leads to frustration, inappropriate services, the potential for medical error and threats to patients' safety, and substantial human and financial costs. Many organizations have attempted to coordinate medical, social, and family resources for these patients, under the premise that doing so will improve their quality of life while reducing medical expenses (Boult, Kane, and Brown 2000). The care system has become too complex for its users, and the usual encounter between physician and patient regularly overlooks many services that would prevent complications or suffering.

For example, educating patients and families to provide self-care is rarely part of physicians' office practice, but it regularly yields better outcomes and lower costs (Lorig et al. 1999). Teaching self-care in classes seems to be more effective than one-on-one education, and the classes also offer socialization and support; but Medicare will not pay for services provided to multiple beneficiaries at the same time (thus, no coverage for classes). Programs that efficiently connect families and patients with needed services often increase costs, since people benefit from more services, but they more reliably meet patients' needs and usually allow them to function better, with reduced symptoms, fewer exacerbations, and otherwise better outcomes.

Geriatric evaluation and management combine evaluation of an older person's medical, psychosocial, and functional capabilities over several months of treatment and follow-up conducted by an interdisciplinary team (at least a doctor, nurse, and social worker) using standardized assessment and treatment protocols. A recent randomized trial showed that geriatric evaluation and management preserved out-patients' functional ability, decreased depressive symptoms, improved satisfaction, and reduced the burden felt by family caregivers, at a cost of about $1,250 per person (Province et al. 1995).

There are a few distinctions between care coordination, case management, and disease management. For the most part, case management uses a medical model to focus on a patient's health care and health status and to coordinate a list of covered services, while care coordination focuses on the patient's need for an array of social services in his or her own environment (such as housing needs, income, and social supports) and coordinates a full range of medical and social support services, including those offered by others, in the community, outside the program (Rosenbach and Young 2000).

Whereas case management tends to serve a smaller group of complex, medically or socially vulnerable "high-risk" patients with highly individualized plans of care, disease management tends to serve a larger group of less individualized patients whose main problem is a single chronic disease. Disease management usually targets populations who are costly and have high but modifiable risks of adverse medical outcomes, including patients with chronic heart failure, diabetes, asthma, chronic obstructive pulmonary disease, or end-stage renal disease. These patients generally have similar primary needs, and the program can take a more standardized approach (Chen et al. 2000; Kane and Kane 2001).

Disease management and care-coordination programs also target different populations and must target them carefully. A program that is too inclusive may be unable to provide the level of services necessary to improve patient outcomes or achieve savings equal to the costs of the program. Similarly, a program that targets too narrowly may miss many appropriate patients and not achieve savings equal to the costs of the program. The literature on chronic-care management interventions has shown that the ability of a program to identify those individuals who would benefit from the interventions is crucial to its success (Wilkinson 1996; Medicare Payment Advisory Commission 2003).

Disease management programs work reasonably well with people who can go to the doctor, use the phone, follow instructions, and have only one major illness; but most of those programs have no experience with a person who has multiple illnesses, hearing and mobility deficits, and other social problems. Care coordination and case management can orchestrate existing services, but they cannot engender new ones; these approaches run into gaps when the needed services simply aren't available. As people become more ill and fragile, for example, having medical services at home can be essential. The care coordinator can identify the problem but cannot fill the need. Thus, no program of care coordination, case management, or disease management is reliably able to serve the sickest patients well. An optimal approach would manage diseases by coordinating services and by generating those not now readily available outside hospice, such as in-home physician care.

Kaiser Permanente's medical center in Bellflower, California, has developed a model program (mentioned earlier) that blends features of these models for patients with heart failure or emphysema (www .growthhouse.org/palliative; Lynn, Nolan, et al. 2002). Since 1995, the program has relied on a nurse practitioner to train patients and families on monitoring symptoms at home to reduce exacerbations and unnecessary hospitalizations. Ties to the Kaiser home health and hospice program have improved care for patients who are nearing the end of life. The program has decreased hospitalizations and increased hospice enrollment for patients with advanced heart and lung disease, patients who are not typically referred to hospice (National Coalition for Health Care and Institute for Healthcare Improvement 2000).

Various studies have indicated that caregivers and care-management clients experience a higher quality of life, have better mental functioning, and enjoy increased social activities. While case management often produces beneficial outcomes for patients, the evidence on the net cost of these programs is mixed (Wilkinson 1996; Boult, Kane, and Brown 2000). Many programs increase the cost of medical care. Case management usually increases spending on community services too. Even so, reduced use of nursing homes may eventually yield net savings, though care-management enrollees are not likely to move to nursing homes soon after enrollment. For these more moderately frail clients, costs are unlikely to be reduced (Wilkinson 1996). Medicare has offered a few demonstration projects to test disease management and the benefit structure that would support it (Crippen 2002; Berenson and Horvath 2003), and the 2003 Medicare reform statute provides for large-scale implementation and evaluation (Medicare Prescription Drug, Improvement, and Modernization Act 2003).

Quality Improvement

Recognizing the shortcomings in end-of-life care, many organizations have undertaken rapid-cycle quality improvement (Phillips, Sabatino, and Long 2001; Lynn, Nolan, et al. 2002). Almost one hundred organizations from an array of health-care facilities and programs have participated in year-long improvement collaboratives. In 1997, forty-seven teams representing hospitals, nursing homes, and veterans hospitals joined in a "Breakthrough Series Collaborative" to improve four key aspects of end-of-life care: to improve pain and other symptom management; to reduce the number of transfers and increase continuity of care; to improve advance care planning; and to attend to the spiritual needs of patients and enhance opportunities for meaningfulness in their lives and in the lives of their loved ones (Lynn, Schuster, and Kabcenell 2000). The forty-seven teams were successful in most of the initiatives that they attempted, although improving continuity of care proved to be a difficult task.

When the collaborative series began, participating teams reported significant problems in how their institutions dealt with end-of-life care (Lynn, Schuster, and Kabcenell 2000). One hospice found that half of the patients it admitted reported pain scores greater than five (on a scale of one to ten). A hospital team found that it took almost an hour from the time pain was assessed until orders were issued and another 115 minutes before medication was actually delivered.

By applying rapid-cycle improvement methods, groups reversed these and other problems. For instance, many teams began to assess pain as a fifth vital sign, a strategy that has since become part of JCAHO standards (Joint Commission on Accreditation of Healthcare Organizations 2001). One team developed what I earlier called the "no surprise" question. The team asked physicians at a Franciscan Health System clinic in Tacoma, Washington, to review lists of their patients—and ask themselves if they would be surprised if particular patients were to die within the next year. Patients whose death would not be a surprise were referred to supportive-care services, including advance care planning. Doing this eventually led to greater satisfaction, more use of supports in the community, earlier referrals to hospice, and much longer stays in hospice care. The program has already expanded to six other facilities in that health-care system and won a national award for its efforts (National Coalition for Health Care and Institute for Healthcare Improvement 2000).

Another team launched an in-patient palliative-care unit in its city's public hospital. That award-winning program relied on community and faith-based volunteer networks to support patients who would otherwise have been ineligible for hospice services (Last Acts 2000).

Building on the success of this model, the U.S. Department of Veterans Affairs, the Institute for Healthcare Improvement, and the Center to Improve Care of the Dying cosponsored a program focused on improving care for patients with advanced congestive heart failure and chronic obstructive pulmonary disease. Regional collaboratives in New York City and in Pittsburgh have demonstrated that the model can be used to move an entire region to improve care for people near the end of life. The Veterans Health System coordinated a quality-improvement collaborative among seventy teams, which drove serious pain rates down by one-third (Cleeland et al. 2003). In these and other projects (Bookbinder 2001), the methods of quality improvement have shown their merit in creating systems that support good care (Lynn, Nolan, et al. 2002; Joint Commission on Accreditation of Healthcare Organizations 2001).

Caregiver Programs

Those aiming to improve end-of-life care increasingly recognize the need to support family (sometimes called "informal") caregivers. Programs aimed at caregivers facing end-of-life issues have yet to be widely developed, although some promising ideas have been proposed or are just getting under way. The National Family Caregiver Support Program, which received congressional funding of $155.2 million in 2003 (Administration on Aging 2003), has allocated funding to provide respite care for family caregivers. Many national organizations, such as the National Alliance for Caregiving and the Family Caregiver Alliance, provide resources and referrals for family caregivers.

California has a statewide program of caregiver resource centers (CRCs) that serve families and caregivers of cognitively impaired adults. This model system gives caregivers a way to access almost all available services that they might need: information, consultations, support, and training. The aim throughout is to reinforce the caregivers' ability to provide and manage needed care. Moreover, the centers integrate their services within existing programs and coordinate among them. This makes a more reliable system for family caregivers, and they are measurably more comfortable with the service system and more satisfied with services that are actually utilized (Friss 1993).

Hospitals are recognizing the important role of caregivers in caring for the chronically ill. The United Hospital Fund supported an initiative in seven hospitals in New York City that aimed to respond more effectively to the needs of family caregivers during and after hospitalization of their sick relatives. Including family caregivers as participants and explicit beneficiaries of planning was regularly possible, and implementation shows that hospitals could shape the caregiving experience. The engagement of caregivers helped mobilize reforms in care processes as well (Levine 2003).

Practice Guidelines and Audit Tools

A few initiatives have aimed to establish standards of practice for those who are very old and/or very sick. For example, the Assessing Care of Vulnerable Elders (ACOVE) Project convened an expert panel of physicians to develop a set of evidence-based quality indicators for vulnerable elders (Wenger, Shekelle, and the ACOVE Investigators 2001). Vulnerable elderly were defined as those older than sixty-five, living in the community, and at high risk for functional decline or death. The project identified end-of-life care as a priority concern (Wenger and Rosenfeld 2001) and developed indicators for discussing and documenting surrogate decision makers, patient-care preferences, and advance directives, as well as for starting and documenting treatments to relieve shortness of breath, pain, and spiritual distress. The panel recommended the use of these quality indicators to compare the care provided by different health-care delivery systems and to evaluate changes over time or in response to intervention. The ACOVE investigators have shown that their measures of quality are met only about half the time (Wenger et al. 2003).

The Last Acts project, a national program office for the Robert Wood Johnson Foundation's projects to improve end-of-life care, convened a palliative-care task force, which promulgated "Precepts of Palliative Care" as the basis for needed reforms (Last Acts 1997). Those precepts call for respect for patients' goals and choices, comprehensive caring services, interdisciplinary teamwork, support for caregivers, and systems capable of supporting good care. Similarly, fifteen professional organizations have signed a statement of core principles for end-of-life care (Cassel and Foley 1999), and Last Acts compiled more than seventy statements on end-of-life care issues by more than forty organizations (Phillips, Sabatino, and Long 2001).

Guidelines for palliative care and pain management have been developed and used to improve end-of-life care. The American Pain Society promoted the concept of pain as a fifth vital sign, which has been widely

adopted (American Pain Society 1995). JCAHO has added this assessment to its standards, and pain is now routinely assessed at hospitals nationwide. In 1999, the Veterans Health Administration added pain assessment to its vital sign assessments (Lynch Schuster 1999). The
veterans program also launched extensive training programs to implement good practices (Veterans Affairs 2002). The American Geriatrics
Society developed guidelines for the management of persistent pain in
older adults (American Geriatrics Society 1997). One study found that
the use of a specific treatment plan for pain management, based on published guidelines, improved patients' pain outcomes. The study's Cancer
Pain Algorithm addresses pain assessment and reassessment, along with
decisions on analgesic drug choice. Its information package includes
comprehensive side-effect protocols, equi-analgesic conversion charts,
and a primer for intractable pain (Du Pen et al. 1999).

Two settings of care that may well have special importance in building good programs of care are nursing homes and managed-care organizations. Nursing homes already provide care for one-quarter of
Medicare decedents, and some contend that this is likely to be half
of all decedents by 2020 (Teno 2003; Brock and Foley 1998). Some
nursing-home improvement projects have reported substantial gains
(Tuch, Parrish, and Romer 2003), and Medicare's quality-improvement
organizations have launched major collaborative quality-improvement
projects on preventing pressure ulcers and pain. Palliative care seems
likely to be a strong development in nursing facilities; a set of guidelines
specifically drawn up for nursing facilities influences that work (Mezey
et al. 2001).

Capitated health-care delivery is another locus of potential ferment
and innovation. Teams like the Kaiser Bellflower team described earlier
have documented substantial gains. Guidelines have been established to
direct improvement activities as managed-care organizations focus upon
end-of-life care (National Task Force on End-of-Life Care in Managed
Care 1999).

Gems and Strategies for Change

A growing number of provider programs are gaining recognition for exceptional work to improve end-of-life care. The American Hospital Association's Circle of Life awards have recognized thirty-five programs that have developed innovations in improving end-of-life care for patients in a broad range of ages, settings, and strategies. One was the hospice program at the Louisiana State Penitentiary at Angola, the largest maximum-security prison in the country, where most of the inmates are serving life sentences. With this innovative hospice program, inmates dying in the prison hospital are able to spend more time with family, be comforted by specially trained inmate volunteers, and receive pain management (*Innovations in End-of-Life Care* 2000).

Other leadership programs have received recognition. The National Coalition for Health Care published a monograph characterizing nine public and private programs that not only provide some component of exemplary care for fatal chronic illness but also measure results and focus on continuous improvement (National Coalition for Health Care and Institute for Healthcare Improvement 2000). The Milbank Memorial Fund and the Robert Wood Johnson Foundation published "Pioneer Programs in Palliative Care: Nine Case Studies" (2000), case studies of the history and characteristics of pioneering palliative-care programs in a common format. The National Hospice and Palliative Care Organization paired up with CAPC to author guidance for hospital-hospice partnerships (Center to Advance Palliative Care 2000b; National Hospice and Palliative Care Organization and Center to Advance Palliative Care 2001). Gradually, guidelines and guidance on pain, advance care planning, palliative-care consultation, and family support are becoming widely available.

Through the program called Community-State Partnerships to Improve End-of-Life Care, twenty-one states and regions have developed community-based initiatives to improve end-of-life care (Midwest Bioethics Center 2002). Activities include developing commissions and task forces to address end-of-life concerns; improving palliative care; establishing quality standards for care in nursing homes and other institutions that care for dying patients; and fostering cooperation and coordination among care providers, including emergency service workers and rescue squads. Another Robert Wood Johnson Foundation project, Promoting Excellence in End-of-Life Care, funded twenty-two grantees nationwide whose demonstration projects aimed at improving care for special populations (such as women, minorities), particular diseases (end-state renal failure, Alzheimer's), and challenging environments (nursing homes, dialysis centers, and jails and prisons) (Promoting Excellence in End-of-Life Care 2002).

The Department of Veterans Affairs accomplished substantial gains through an initiative focused on end-of-life and palliative care, which included measurable performance and a small bonus tied to accomplishment. VA Faculty Leaders Project for Improved Care at the End of Life helped thirty internal medicine residency programs to develop benchmark curricula for end-of-life and palliative medicine (Veterans Health Care System 2002). The success of this work evolved into a fellowship program for physicians, nurses, and other health-care professionals in hospice and palliative care. By 2004, every Veterans Medical Center had a clinical service in palliative care.

In sum, illuminating and vigorous forays into system reform are already occurring, but most are underfunded, short-term, and limited in scope. The next phase of innovation and evaluation might well involve more sizable changes and more enduring strategies for change. The pilots and innovations so far have shown that most patients can manage much of their care and plan ahead, that most symptoms can be prevented or relieved, and that many malfunctions in the care system can be overcome, at least some of the time.

In Britain, Progress in Care for the Last Part of Life
Joanne Lynn

When considering a set of issues like care for the last part of life, one reasonably assumes that other countries have important insights and working programs that might guide and inspire reform activities in the United States. After all, every demographically similar nation faces roughly the same challenges—long-term illness at the end of life, projected growth of the affected population, and social arrangements that reflect an earlier era dominated by acute illnesses. Indeed, many innovations and advances are in evidence. Hospice programs are available around the world (www.iahpc.org), Canada has promulgated a substantial set of standards and has designated specific funds for end-of-life care, and the World Health Organization (2004) has issued guidance for palliative care.

As one might expect, since the modern movement for palliative care started there with the work of Cicely Saunders (Saunders and Clark 2002), Britain often leads the way in implementing better care for the last phase of life. A major difference in the British approach to reform, as compared to that in the United States, is that the care system has authorities that can shape its evolution. Each area has its Strategic Health Authority, Hospital Trust, Primary Care Trust, facilities, staff, and governing leadership. When these authorities are most concerned with defending the status quo, they can block innovation. But when they are forward-looking and invested in improvement, they can create engines of reform quickly. At present, the tenor of such efforts seems to be looking to improve care toward the end of life, sponsoring widespread innovation, measurement of accomplishments, and investment in better ways to organize care.

Britain has a reinvention project for its National Health Service (NHS) generally, and that modernization agenda has included end-of-life care from the start. Led by Dr. Keri Thomas, the British Gold Standards Framework has engaged more than one-tenth of the General Practitioners in activities that demonstrably improve care, including having a registry of persons sick enough to die, ensuring that these patients and families have adequate support at home after office hours, documenting where each person wants to be when near death, and trying to effectuate that wish (keri .thomas@btinternet.com; www.goldstandardsframework.nhs.uk). The British National Institute for Clinical Excellence is responsible for documenting guidelines to achieve high quality, and guidelines for palliative care are in place alongside those for many other aspects of health care (National Institute for Clinical Excellence 2003; www.nice.org.uk). Over time, these will be part of the regulatory reviews and the bonus payments for high performance. The guidelines specifically endorse the Gold Standards Framework and also the Liverpool Care Pathway (www.lcp-mariecurie.org.uk), a checklist of issues to address in order to ensure reliable support near the end of life (Macmillan Cancer Relief 2004).

Britain has also developed extensive and reasonably comprehensive care arrangements, including in-patient hospice services, able to serve virtually every community. Those hospice programs have become major providers of expertise to hospitals and other providers. Britain has established a specialty in palliative medicine, requiring certified training in order to practice as a palliative-care physician. Each geographic area has a District Nurse home-care service and a Macmillan cancer home-care nursing service, and these programs have undertaken additional training for many of these nurses.

Increasingly, the British health-care system believes that moving patients into the hospital near death serves neither the patients nor the care system well. More than half of all deaths in Britain take place in a hospital. Part of the Gold Standards Framework requires documenting the patient's preferred place of care at the end of life and following that preference whenever possible. More District Nurses and General Practitioners are able to support family caregiving at home, and family caregivers usually qualify for a stipend from the government. In addition, enhancing nursing-home capabilities for adequate care has become a priority.

Continuity across care settings and time has been a challenge and will be even more complicated when the new contract with General Practitioners takes effect in 2004, since the new contract eliminates any requirement to take after-hours calls. The Primary Care Trusts that manage primary care will need to devise ways to ensure that after-hours on-call teams know each patient's situation and are able to respond to the home if needed. Electronic medical records, which are beginning to be widely implemented, will help with this challenge. In part because care is often compartmentalized in a series of settings and in part because the care system is less driven by legal considerations, advance care planning has not been as substantial a focus in Britain as it has in the United States. The growing requirement to know the preferred place of care may well spur a broader consideration of preferences and options.

4

SURVEYING THE TERRAIN

Opportunities and Challenges

Eventually, good care will require major changes in our culture—the way we structure reality, what facts we take to be salient, and the language we use. Indeed, I judge that most of these cultural changes are largely inevitable—what well-considered strategy can do is to accelerate the pace of change and avoid inept care and suffering for many as we undertake reforms.

This chapter lays out a number of approaches to the entrenched barriers I foreshadow above, as well as arguments for focusing upon caregivers and financing and high-leverage opportunities for change. Some of my claims will be controversial, not only to those who have not yet endorsed the need for substantial reforms in care for people in the last years of life but also among those who work in palliative care, long-term care, and elder services. A productive, ongoing public discussion would help shape and galvanize support for a useful agenda.

The prospects for social reforms always depend upon our specific situation—the challenges and opportunities that our particular history and situation engender. Reformers must create and implement strategic plans; it is always difficult to gauge whether any particular strategy might be suitable for implementation and what effects it would actually have. Very experienced and insightful strategists are often proven wrong. But by thinking through the situation, considering a range of alternative actions, and judging the likely course and effects of each, we can argue for putting efforts toward the highest-leverage actions rather than pursuing opportunities as they happen to come up.

I have become convinced that no individual patients or physicians and nurses—however beneficent their actions—can resolve the issues in care for the last phase of life. Of course, activated patients and skillful clinicians are going to do better than others; but the dysfunctions are so widespread and so intrinsic to the care arrangements that major reforms at the organizational or political levels will be essential.

Key Features of Change

Fundamentally, major social change requires convergence of a number of forces that make the old way of doing things untenable while making a new order appealing or at least necessary. As we survey the structures for care of those with serious chronic illnesses, some of the facts seem especially salient. First, long-term disability and care needs in the years before dying do not generate large profits or attract substantial investments. Most of the patients are poor already or fear becoming poor. Most of the services involve low-paid labor, performed by those with limited political influence. The major sources of revenue for health-care providers are medications, devices, and hospitalizations, many of which are subject to inappropriate overuse now and are often hard to justify in a more ideal care delivery system (Fisher et al. 2003a; Fisher et al. 2003b). Most public policy makers and leaders—in academia or health systems, or in pharmaceuticals or technical applications—do not yet see reforms for serious chronic illness care as particularly attractive, or even important.

Second, while there have been a few important innovations (some characterized in chapter 3), they have been neither so widely attempted nor so well studied as to provide a sure guide. Beyond hospices, we mostly have small or thinly supported innovations. We have almost no study of the trade-offs among modes of care. The data on family caregiving, its effects, and alternatives are so fragmented as to be misleading. We urgently need innovations and the insights gained from testing them. We must begin to try new methods of care delivery, along with new mental models, ethics, politics, social roles, and figures of speech.

Third, the political weight for reforms cannot come just from the palliative-care providers; our numbers are too small and our influence is too limited. Indeed, the hard scramble for initial successes has fragmented the forces of hospice, long-term care, palliative care, PACE, and others, leaving them little tradition of aligning to pursue common goals.

As we look about for allies who might have the authority to garner political weight, we cannot count on those living now with serious and eventually fatal chronic illnesses in the last part of their lives, those most directly affected by the challenges of our care system. Overwhelming personal issues make it unlikely that they will seek attention within the political process. Even when they do raise their claims, they will not necessarily be alive through the next elections. Those who will face the issues in a few years, either when their parents become ill or when they do, are not yet engaged.

Yet all those currently struggling with the inadequacies of care in the last phase of life have families and other caregivers. That's where the political clout could lie—with all of the baby boomers who will first take care of their parents and then see their own suffering looming in the disarray and dysfunction of the care "system." The boomers have a long history of "having it their way" in politics. Perhaps, as caregivers, they could mobilize to fix the shortcomings before it becomes their turn to be the patients.

Reformers and allies should advocate for a reliable, sustainable approach to competent care for the large population of people seriously affected by eventually fatal chronic conditions. For this part of life, the care system should function differently. Often, everything that matters in the life left to such individuals hinges on the care arrangements being effective in providing supportive services. Symptom control, family support, continuity of a comprehensive care plan, and counseling for life closure will need to be reliably competent across a variety of settings. Hence, the metric by which to measure success will be more complicated than the traditional measure of quality—delay of death.

The delivery of care will have to change, along with its financing. Improved delivery arrangements and enhanced financing must mesh, since no clinical-care system lasts long if it cannot pay its bills. Conversely, more tailored financing cannot be much ahead of clinical reforms, because dysfunctional adaptations by providers arise quickly to respond to business opportunities and then defend against further reforms that would disadvantage that business plan.

More than four of every five Americans die while covered by Medicare—and many while also covered by Medicaid. The obvious "hammer" for the financing "nail" is the existing federal financing of care delivery, along with a number of derivative endeavors in regulation, human resource development, and law. The public truly owns this care system.

The clinical reforms needed to match improved financing can arise from a larger variety of sources. The anchor could be hospice programs, since hospice is available virtually everywhere in the country. However, advocates for primary care (internal medicine, family practice, and advanced practice nursing) and geriatric interdisciplinary teamwork may well step forward, aware that care of the very sick at home is powerfully satisfying. Nursing facilities will undoubtedly be the residence of many of us in our last months, so enhanced care in that setting will be important. The unusual combination of flexible financing and the needy populations served by PACE and the Veterans Health System may well make them ongoing loci of innovation and setting standards. In summary, the main financing reform has to be Medicare and Medicaid payment policy, but the improved clinical services can arise from various existing providers.

In addition to the obvious challenges of major Medicare and Medicaid reforms, a series of troubling quandaries at the boundary of ethics and policy cramps our efforts to leverage change: our inability to temper the use of high-cost medical treatments that have modest merit in extending life; our uncertainty as to appropriate care for persons with substantial dementia or other brain damage; and the threats of liability and human subjects protections that serve to retard innovation.

Caregivers as a Political Force

The growing numbers of very sick, older people coming to the ends of their lives and the declining numbers of people available to provide direct care create a looming disproportion that presents both a critical challenge and a major opportunity. If very sick and disabled people cannot have competent and caring day-to-day personal assistance, then almost everything else we could have at that phase of life is also largely unobtainable. Without caregivers, nearly all of us, in our turn, will endure otherwise quite avoidable suffering.

Changes in the living conditions of very sick people sometimes ease their need for care. When the Social Security Administration started sending monthly checks directly to banks, many people who previously answered surveys by saying that they needed help with managing financial matters now found they could handle their finances on their own. As housing gradually becomes more adapted to suit people with disabilities, more people will be able to manage getting to the toilet from their wheelchairs; and as more areas have home delivery of groceries, more people will be able to manage to prepare food. These gains are likely to be limited, since many people have disabilities beyond those that these adaptations can circumvent and since the adaptations themselves can be too costly. The burgeoning numbers of people facing progressive chronic illnesses will still need care, so the focus will have to be upon adding to the supply of caregivers. Four approaches seem plausible:

- Increase the numbers of reliable paid caregivers for home and nursing home (mainly aides and nurses).
- Improve the availability and reliability of informal (family, unpaid) caregiving.
- Expand both the quantity and quality of caregiving in communities (including by religious organizations and neighbors).
- Provide or substitute for some personal-care services using machines or trained animals.

The first approach, making more paid caregivers available, does have promise. Paid caregivers usually earn just above the minimum wage, which is well below the level necessary to support a family. The conditions of their work—at times in cramped apartments up many flights of stairs or in suburban homes far from public transportation—can be wearing; the job itself is difficult and often thankless; patients may be unable or unwilling to show appreciation. Often, friction arises as patients find the need for help embarrassing and frustrating and feel very isolated by being homebound or in a nursing home. And the caregiver's native language and culture often differ from the patient's. In addition, most working situations offer little chance for advancement, further training, or better working conditions.

The opportunities for improving this picture are obvious. Just extending employment benefits for health-care insurance and disability income support would enhance the likelihood that skilled caregivers will enter and stay in the field. Increasing wages and incorporating caregivers into larger health-care teams would create more appealing and honored positions (Callahan 2001). Well-considered training opportunities and career ladders would probably help too. Of course, these changes have costs, but so does the hospitalization or high-cost treatment they may allow a patient to avoid.

Unpaid family caregivers encounter additional challenges. For example, family caregivers contend with thoroughly unfamiliar situations and would benefit from improved training and support to learn essential caregiving skills (such as how to give a bed bath, set up oxygen, and so on; recall Carol Levine's saga, following chapter 1). These caregivers also need protection from severe financial burdens arising from lost current income and retirement savings. Paying for their services at a discounted rate and providing pension contributions are approaches used in some European countries (Merlis 2000). Providing protection against reduced retirement benefits via Social Security and pension arrangements would help. Family caregivers also need ways to pursue some of their personal life goals—through regular outside help or occasional respite care, for example.

It would undoubtedly help too if society valued family caregiving and respected the people who do this hard work. Since family caregivers are serving the community, that community should ensure that caregivers have jobs when they are ready to return to work, health and disability insurance throughout their time of service, the ability to save money for retirement, and approval and collegiality from their community. Family caregivers warrant the kind of respect that society accords to others who do good works as a service to the community, much as reservists in the National Guard have some employment guarantees and benefits. In our present circumstances, we have allowed it to be very hard to be a family caregiver—no training, pay, job security, insurance, pension, or even thanks from the community. At least the current situation presents many opportunities for improvement.

The public costs of supporting family caregivers may turn out to be a good investment in enhancing care and avoiding the costs of institutionalization. For example, I have estimated the likely annual cost of a statute to allow otherwise uninsured caregivers fifty-five to sixty-four years of age to buy into Medicare without paying extra for preexisting conditions. For less than $200 million per year, we would cover an especially vulnerable group of people who need health care themselves (and who often can't reenter the job market when direct caregiving ends because of their own existing health conditions). This kind of strategy would be a visible way to honor and encourage family caregiving.

The use of robotic machines and specially trained animals may seem unrealistic, or at least futuristic, but many chores might well be automated or carried out by companion animals. Computers with video teleconferencing capabilities can monitor the needs of frail elderly. Lifts that help move patients, telephones that respond to vocal signals, lights that turn on with movement, and alerting devices that monitor vital signs all aid in relieving some of the burden of home-care workers and in providing a sense of independence to patients (Mann 2001). Priorities for development of new devices might include better ways to reduce pressure and increase mobility and thereby prevent pressure ulcers, to move and transfer people, and to automate the supervision of people who cannot exercise judgment. Developing these possibilities is important, though neither machines nor service animals should displace human interaction and caring.

The following specific reforms would improve the availability and working conditions of caregivers:

- Provide health, disability, and retirement benefits for caregivers, whether they are wage earners or family volunteers.
- Pay professional caregivers a living wage and offer a career ladder for experience and skills.
- Pay family caregivers, at least those with low incomes.
- Encourage family caregiving through graduated tax credits.
- Give all caregivers adequate training and at-home support.
- Enlarge the supportive services of community networks, church-based services, and other local groups.
- Invest in developing machinery and trained animals for some tasks.
- Encourage respect for hands-on caregivers and awareness of their role and value by publicizing accounts of their work.

Making caregiving more bearable, and possibly even rewarding, is clearly critical for any reforms to succeed, but another mission makes caregivers especially important: their potential political weight. A very sick person is hardly likely to become a political force. But the family and friends who struggle within the current care system are best able to see the problems and to engage in political activity, either while in the process of caregiving or later. Indeed, family members might even come to voice concerns in political terms in anticipation of caregiving, as the shortcomings of patient care and caregiver support become more widely known. Usually, family caregivers see their problems as intimate and unique. They are unaware that the dysfunctions are systematic, that they belong to a class of people who all have the same problems, and that better legislation, regulation, and social arrangements could lighten their burden. In this case, the personal is truly political, and caregivers could become an important force in the court of public opinion.

What would allow us to forge a group consciousness and political agenda for family caregivers? Here are some possibilities:

- Tie family caregivers together by newsletters, on-line conversations, political agendas, and organizations.
- Encourage caregiver organizations to articulate shared agendas.
- Encourage organizations with allied interests, such as disease-based or aging-relevant organizations, to support these issues.
- Push political leadership to articulate positions on caregiver issues.
- Draw in business and employee interests.
- Tell stories of family caregiving in magazines and newspapers and on radio and television.

All reform faces substantial challenges from inertia, as well as special challenges from the specifics of a particular time and place. The shortage of potential caregivers provides both a powerful motivation and a daunting challenge for any future care arrangements. This predictable need and the problems in providing for it may well be the most powerful motivation for change. As Rosalynn Carter has said, "There are only four kinds of people in the world: those who have been caregivers, those who are currently caregivers, those who will be caregivers, and those who need caregiving" (Rosalynn Carter Institute for Human Development 2003). Recognizing this truth may make a broad cross section of citizens into a political force for reform, once people with each of these four perspectives on being a family caregiver realize that political action is essential to address our shared problems.

The Business Case for Change

In the current system, federal policy shapes care for the last phase of life, because federal dollars pay for most of the health-care costs incurred at that time. Yet there is no coherent agenda, and no federal agency monitors and addresses the needs and priorities of this part of life. Although payment and coverage policies generally ensure ready access to surgery, diagnostic tests, and physician-directed treatments, they do not cover continuity of care over the long term, home health care, symptom control, and family and caregiver support. Many of the most successful programs for people living with eventually fatal chronic diseases are directed by nurses or social workers, serve patients in classrooms and at home, ensure that medications are available, and are dedicated to good advance care planning. But Medicare does not generally cover these services and strategies. Indeed, Medicare's payment policies yield no workable business plan for physicians and hospitals that aim to provide coordinated and comprehensive care to those who face serious chronic illnesses (Lynn, Wilkinson, and Etheredge 2001).

Medicare has certainly been one of the valued legacies of the idealism and social reform of mid-twentieth-century America (Stevens 1996). For nearly forty years, the United States has ensured that its elderly can count on medical care. The population's needs have changed over time, and, as the aging population grows, so will its needs for care. Since Medicare's passage, pressures for change have mostly come from providers interested in defending their opportunities (for example, pursuing improved payment rates), from groups advocating coverage of those with particular diseases, or in reaction to rising aggregate costs. These agendas do not address the reliability and quality of service. Reformers will face challenges in finding politically powerful ways to bring quality and reliability to center stage.

In our present situation, a major risk to the well-being of those coming to the end of life is that the generally unreliable care for those who

are old and sick will become so costly and so broadly mistrusted that thi, society will renege on its commitment to their care. Some experts insist that the commitment has actually been fairly fragile throughout Medicare's history (Marmor 2000). If the care is not trustworthy and the body politic decides that the costs are unbearable, it may well retreat from the current broad commitment to health care for the elderly to a political solution that effectively makes each person responsible for finding and funding his or her own services. Not only would that be inequitable, it would ensure ongoing failure in the delivery of services. No one person can generate a good disease management program for advanced heart failure—such programs are feasible only if they enroll almost every heart failure patient in a region. Thinking that each sick and dying person can shop for services is like expecting individuals to shop around and pay only for the roads they want. Some services simply are not likely to be broadly available and of high quality unless leaders organize them to serve a population. Yet vouchers and other forms of limiting both the commitment to the elderly and the moral responsibility of providers have a real political seductiveness and an existing constituency (Cook 1999).

Building a reliable care array that people value and trust and that engenders only a sustainable cost is the best available pathway toward sustaining the historic community commitment to health care for the elderly. The main financing mechanism for medical services in the last phase of life is Medicare, which covers 83 percent of all who die in the United States (Hogan et al. 2000). Medicare mostly pays fee-for-service, with 92 percent of beneficiaries having this "traditional Medicare" at the time of death. In this coverage arrangement, doctors, hospitals, and other providers of service are paid for each billed service, though hospitalization itself is mostly paid with one fee for the entire hospitalization. Fee-for-service payment encourages billable services, but not continuity. (A particularly striking example of the distortions this payment mechanism generates is described in the next section of this chapter.) No coverage is

ordinarily available for caregiver training, classroom education of patients, on-call advice, bereavement, or spiritual counseling, so they are effectively discouraged.

The Medicare+Choice part of Medicare (now renamed Medicare Advantage) is "managed care," which pays on a per-month capitated rate. This per-patient, per-month payment allows the program to be more flexible in tailoring services, but adverse incentives remain. In Medicare managed care, the rates do not reflect the severity of illness. Adjustments in rate for diagnoses that caused hospitalization now apply, but those adjustments do not reflect the differences in costs between caring for persons with early illness and caring for those with advanced illness. Capitated programs, therefore, do better financially if they sign up and keep only relatively healthy patients; they cannot afford a good reputation for care of the very sick. Thus, while advertisements on buses tout health-care plans' successes with injuries and immunizations, no advertising placard lures those who are already very sick with progressive chronic conditions.

Payments in the Veterans Health Care System are budgeted and salaried, and that may be part of the reason that the veterans system has been a leader in improving care for serious chronic illness and the end of life. Serving patients correctly does not financially disadvantage any veterans' provider. But the Veterans Health Care System as a whole is thinly funded, a situation that may limit the sustainability of its gains.

Payments in hospice and PACE are capitated, usually at a rate that more closely matches service needs. Some of the good reputation of hospice and PACE may well have its origin in their more adequate and more flexible funding, as well as their targeted services and selected population.

Overall, though, the payment for medical services to most who live out the end of life covered by Medicare does not match service needs closely. Services for long-term care at home or in a nursing home are fragmented, highly regulated, inadequately paid, and often undesirable in quality. Even worse, about half of the costs of care for those in their last year or two arises from long-term care or prescription drugs. Medicare has not generally covered these (Maxwell, Moon, and Segal

2001). The financing arrangements are regularly impoverishing to patients who need long-term care, whether at home or in a facility. Medicare covers only a small proportion of long-term care, since most comes from personal assets or, when the person is seriously impoverished, Medicaid. The rates Medicaid pays approximate the lowest that the community can pay without creating scandalous conditions. For supportive services such as nursing-home care, Medicaid routinely sets the rate below actual care needs, and substantial improvements often come only with evidence of widespread inadequate care. In contrast, the health care that generates substantial financial returns tends to be drugs, devices, and technology-dependent procedures; and the costs in development, delivery, and profit for these are built into the price. Sadly, neither kind of rate setting establishes incentives for quality and efficiency.

In Washington, D.C., many Medicaid-dependent nursing-home residents need 4.0 hours a day of in-person direct care; Medicaid rates support, at best, about 2.5 hours. Fairly predictably, our city council holds hearings about the scandalous conditions of care in nursing homes. How the financing runs, how much money aides make, and how much care residents need are not prominent topics. This political drama is commonplace in most states. State budgets cannot readily accommodate escalating payments, so the focus is often just on regulations and penalties. While this complex interaction has heroes and villains on all sides, my point here is only that the community does have a stake in having reliable and efficient nursing-home care, and perhaps this, too, can become a positive political agenda, pushed by a self-interested populace.

Clearly, the incentives and coverage throughout the last phase of life are adverse to patients' interests in counting on good care. What would be better?

· Criteria for performance—continuity, symptom relief, advance
   care planning, and other important elements of care—could influence payment.

- Options of salaried, budgeted, or capitated payment would allow flexibility and reduce dysfunctional incentives.
- The costs of providing appropriate services could determine payment.

Since each of these strategies still has substantial adverse incentives, a blend of strategies might well work best.

Promoting Coordinated Care— A Potential Anchor of Major Reform

How serious is the claim that incentives are misaligned? A few years ago, I worked out the finances of a particularly commonplace example: care of a person with frailty and serious chronic heart failure. The ways to optimize care for patients with "bad pumps" are well known. More than a dozen well-designed and published studies (Rich et al. 1995; Phillips et al. 2004) show that early intervention at the first sign of fluid retention, optimal diet and medication, and gentle exercise greatly reduce the use of hospitals. Indeed, most patients use hospitals less than half as often in a program of coordinated care as they do with uncoordinated care from an ordinary doctor's office. In teams that add advance care planning for the end of life and rapid response to the home for any worsening of symptoms, the rate of use of emergency rooms can go down to one-tenth of the prior rate (Lynn, Schall, et al. 2000). Table 3 tallies the costs of providing services, the Medicare payments, and the net income to providers in two scenarios of care for a typical elderly couple, whose possible stories follow.

Case Study

Ordinary course of care

Mary Smith, seventy-eight years old, had osteoporosis, diabetes mellitus, mild heart failure, and cataracts at the time of her diagnosis with breast cancer.

Her husband, eighty-four, had cognitive impairment and, since having a stroke, was dependent upon her for transfers, bathing, and dressing. They lived on a small pension in a rented apartment. Their children lived at a distance, and the Smiths had few contacts except for health care. During the turmoil and financial challenges of his wife's cancer treatments, Mr. Smith's condition worsened, and he entered a nursing home. Mrs. Smith wore herself out with worry, and her heart failure worsened. Her husband died of a urinary tract infection in a hospital intensive-care unit. Mrs. Smith developed back pain and constipation but would not go to her physician's office for an evaluation. Eventually she became delirious and was admitted to the hospital as an emergency patient. She could not keep her apartment and entered a nursing home. A few months later, Mrs. Smith also died in the hospital, after being transferred because of pulmonary edema. Through all this, the couple had much suffering, a dozen different physicians, and several hospitalizations (and, for each, death in the hospital).

Better course of care

As soon as Mary Smith was diagnosed with cancer, her physician recognized that the Smiths' situation was rife with risks. He involved a nurse care coordinator who worked with the couple through the rest of their lives, planning ahead and marshaling needed services in a timely way. The care coordinator contacted the church the Smiths had attended and elicited some friendly visitors and volunteer help. The city provided in-home aides and repair services to enable them to stay in their apartment, even when chemotherapy left Mrs. Smith fatigued. When Mr. Smith had another stroke, a home-care program helped for a few weeks until he died at home. Suffering from heart failure, Mrs. Smith had more trouble with shopping and housework, so she moved to senior apartments that provided meal and maid service. She died in her sleep quietly one night.

Adapted from Lynn J, Wilkinson A, Etheredge L. 2001. Financing of care for fatal chronic disease: opportunities for Medicare reform. *West J Med.* 175:299–302. With permission from the BMJ Publishing Group.

Table 3. *How the money moves*

	Ordinary Care (U.S. $)			Better Care (U.S. $)		
Service	Production cost	Medicare payment	Provider net income[a]	Production cost	Medicare payment	Provider net income[a]
Home nursing visits	200	210	10	3,000	2,300	(700)
Physician office visits	600	350	(250)	100	120	20
Physician home visits	0	0	0	1,000	450	(550)
Physician hospital visits	2,000	2,300	300	0	0	0
Care coordination	0	0	0	3,000	500	(2,500)
Hospitalizations	20,000	21,000	1,000	0	0	0
ER and ambulance	1,500	2,000	500	0	0	0
Total	24,300	25,860	1,560	7,100	3,370	(3,730)

Source: Adapted from Lynn J, Wilkinson A, Etheredge L. 2001. Financing of care for fatal chronic disease: opportunities for Medicare reform. Table 1. *West J Med.* 175:299–302. With permission from the BMJ Publishing Group.

Note: Amounts are estimated from experience and from published tables of Medicare reimbursements. Estimates exclude costs that are not generally covered by Medicare, such as nursing facility, home health aide, assisted-living facility, and prescription drugs.

[a] Provider net income is the difference between the payments and the costs of production, which include salary costs for the professionals and their practice costs. Numbers in parentheses represent net losses.

Many readers will find the discrepancy in care hard to believe. That's good: it *should* seem astonishing, but it's accurate. Our care system regularly pays more than $25,000 for services that provide emergency care for preventable complications of heart failure, although better care could be had for $8,000. Why aren't doctors and hospitals organizing to provide this better care? Current care arrangements use the services of every type of provider. Hospitals make money, doctors make money, and patients and families are grateful for the rescue services. In better care, with present reimbursement plans, every provider loses money. No one can afford to provide services that regularly lose money. Thus, moving to the improved arrangement faces the certainty of financial disaster, as well as the commonplace resistance to change. Even though the improved practices would do more to relieve suffering and extend life than most drugs and devices for heart failure, which have eager markets, those improved practices are not generally available. Medicare's coverage policies and the necessary self-interest of providers ensure inadequate and costly care.

This gap in practices has been widely known, and managed care, employer-sponsored disease management, and the veterans health system have been able to implement better practices. But fee-for-service Medicare covers the vast majority of people suffering from advanced chronic heart failure, and fee-for-service beneficiaries have usually not been able to have better care. This would seem to offer an opportunity for dramatic improvement that could sweep in larger reforms. Under the Medicare reform statute enacted in 2003, Medicare will pay for disease management services for patients with chronic heart failure, diabetes, and emphysema (Medicare Prescription Drug, Improvement, and Modernization Act of 2003). Payment requires that providers improve quality of care and keep costs low. Organizations that already provide such services must offer patient education and adhere to guidelines for good care. With the elderly, providers will quickly learn that good care also requires developing more comprehensive services, ensuring continuity, and planning ahead. Adapting the new program to meet the needs could provide the opening wedge for major reforms, such as the strategy for care I present in chapter 5.

In summary, reform could build on the opportunity presented by the troubling shortcomings in care for chronic heart failure:

- Highlight the scandalous situation in which the financing and habits of American medicine allow persistently inadequate care, perhaps thereby forging the will to demand reform.
- Rapidly try out and evaluate alternative implementation strategies, to work out specific details of better service delivery and payment arrangements.
- Use the virtually certain success with heart failure to focus attention on the broader population living with eventually fatal chronic illnesses.

Barriers to Reform

Much of the resistance to reform arises from the "usual suspects" of self-interest and inertia among those who make a living under the current arrangements, as well as inattention engendered by a widespread distaste for reminders of implacable mortality. A few issues entail conflicts among deeply held political and ethical values; society's unwillingness to deal with these both obstruct more productive resolutions and set intractable challenges for reform efforts. The three issues that I highlight here are these:

Treatment that is slightly effective but expensive

Treatment that might extend life with dementia

Forces that retard innovation

EFFECTIVE BUT EXPENSIVE TREATMENT

Effective new drugs and devices promise to overwhelm the health-care budget. As just one example among many, the increasing use of implanted cardioverter defibrillators (called ICDs) will generate remarkable expenses within just a few years. Under the restricted criteria from the Multicenter Automatic Defibrillator Implantation Trial II, three or four million Americans already qualify for an implanted defibrillator that can stop most life-ending heart irregularities (Moss et al. 2002). Another six hundred thousand qualify each year. One estimate put the costs per year of life extended at $125,000 (Greene 2000). Each device costs $25,000, and implanting and regulating it cost about that much every year. Even if only the new cases actually got the device, and if life span with the device averages a few years, the costs would be at least $60 billion per year (600,000 people/year × $100,000/person = $60 billion/year). Most of these costs are in Medicare, since the heart condition mostly affects older people. Even with these deliberately conservative estimates, defibrillators would account for one-eighth of the current Medicare budget (Center for Medicare and Medicaid Services 2002)—for a device that was not included in budget projections just a year or two ago. ICDs are effective and, on average, extend life. They also make it much less likely that dying will be sudden. For some patients, the other ways they could die may well be rather more difficult.

This kind of high-cost but effective treatment challenges the social fabric in new ways. Medicare has long been mandated to provide all advantageous treatments that are proven effective for particular conditions. No part of the approval, pricing, or coverage process even allows anyone to make decisions to restrict availability on the basis of costs once the treatment is shown to be more effective than older alternatives. New treatments like defibrillators may finally have brought society to the breaking point. In the 1980s, the nation absorbed the expenses of dialysis and kidney transplants, despite unexpectedly high costs. In comparison with those who could use implantable defibrillators and genetically engineered drugs, the potential pool of renal failure patients was small, and patients were often young and otherwise healthy. The pool of people eligible for the newer developments is much larger, older, and sicker.

While implantable defibrillators are a particularly visible and costly example, many other treatments raise the same questions. Lung volume reduction surgery (http://cms.hhs.gov/ncdr/memo.asp?id = 96), left ventricular assist devices (http://cms.hhs.gov/ncdr/memo.asp?id = 79), and genetically engineered drugs are new entries in the high-cost sweepstakes; but chemotherapy for advanced cancer (Emanuel et al. 2003), intensive-care-unit support for the very old and frail, and expanding use of erythropoetin to stimulate blood production are existing examples of the same widespread use with small gain. Left ventricular assist devices, on average, extend life less than a year at a cost of over $2,500,000 (Gillick 2004). Perhaps even the affected patients might have higher priorities for that sizable fund (Smith et al. 2003).

Talk of "rationing" health care has an ominous ring to the public and, as a result, to politicians. Nevertheless, more treatments now successfully extend life for people who have very limited life spans and life possibilities. All of us, and our political leadership especially, must address questions of balance and merit (Callahan 1998). Failing to do so forces us to go on as we are now—unable to talk about acceptable deaths, extended but undesirable life conditions, or priorities among social investments.

If we cannot limit the distortions possible from providing very high-cost treatments mostly aimed at people in the last tenth of their lives, then we may shave away or deny funding for aides, nurses, housing, and other fundamentals. Denying a particular medication or treatment that patients or families want often proves to be contentious and public. Reducing those services that are hard to track or to demand, or whose benefit is not so dramatically apparent, is much easier. For example, hospices that once provided four to six hours per day of home health aide coverage have gradually cut back to the occasional one- or two-hour session. No one notices this, but families would be up in arms if the hospice instead restricted use of high-cost pain medications. So the challenge now is to establish a method by which the federal budget for care of those with fatal chronic illnesses can match the dominant problems and concerns of patients and families, even if this framework means that very costly treatments are sometimes not readily available to some patients who might benefit.

Accomplishing this aim will be quite difficult in our culture. Americans are proud of making every proven medical treatment available to all, at least in Medicare. Medicare cannot lawfully refuse to cover a treatment because it is costly. The urgent question that these costly treatments set before us is whether the merit for patients is worth the cost to society.

As we try to learn how to generate an answer, what approaches might work better? First, we could tailor services to evidence indicating what the covered population values, allowing for some latitude for patients with unusual preferences. For example, in 2003, geriatricians debated whether residents in nursing homes with modestly elevated lipid profiles should have lipid-lowering drugs, given that new data showed slightly improved survival, even in old age. In the usual course of things, that argument would simply carry the day, and a standard would be set to use lipid-lowering drugs even in advanced old age and even for persons with severe cognitive failure. But such a decision should at least weigh the preferences of the residents, their families, and their hands-on caregivers. At prices in 2003, the costs for a two-hundred-bed nursing home would be about $150,000 per year. Suppose we asked a broad set of those most concerned—the residents, families, and nursing assistants—to list the uses of $150,000 that would enhance the lives of the residents. As it turns out, no one with whom I have discussed this situation believes that affected parties would ever list using the money on lipid-lowering drugs. My point here is that data about the preferences of the parties most affected actually have almost no force in setting the care system's priorities. If we set out to make them salient, we could require evidence of these preferences in coverage decisions and standard setting. While the preferences of individual patients and families should be weighed in individual treatment decisions, I am most interested here in giving the aggregate preferences of affected groups of patients and families a role in shaping the care delivery system. Because not all options are feasible, we would serve patients well if the options that mattered most were also the most readily available.

A second approach would be to find ways to expect or require consideration of coexisting medical problems and shortened life expectancy in decisions about providing treatments. When Medicare considers coverage of implantable defibrillators, as described earlier, the data that policy makers use have evaluated the usefulness of the device in stopping death in people afflicted mostly with heart failure. The study patients must be in good enough health that they are not expected to die of something else in the near future. Yet actual patients ordinarily have other serious illnesses that limit life expectancy. Indeed, patients receiving ICDs are not generally warned that they will want to stop the defibrillator at some point before dying, either to avert the troubling firing of electric shocks when near death or to accept dying of heart rhythm irregularities rather than waiting for another, more difficult, course to death.

TREATMENT OF DEMENTIA

The nature of life with dementia, and the latitude allowed to family choices and advance planning that decide whether or not to treat to extend life, strikes many people as a troubling situation. We want to honor the dignity and worth of all human beings, but we also often find it unacceptable or at least unnecessary to make life longer once dementia has robbed people of their character, memories, and capabilities. While individuals and families struggle with these issues as they play out in a family member, we also need a workable social consensus, and approval of at least an accepted range of options. With half of people who die after age eighty-five having a cognitive deficit (Evans et al. 1989), society will have to make peace with a range of choices about treatments to prolong life with serious and progressive dementia. Indeed, it may be that assessment of people's perceptions of what to value in severe dementia would mostly find priorities of comfort, dignity, cleanliness, skin care, and consideration for a family's burdens—and not prolonged life.

The sentiments embodied in the Americans with Disabilities Act and other public policies to defend the interests of people with disabilities make it difficult for anyone except the affected person to weigh the value of extended life (National Council on Disability 2003). If a person with a particular medical problem and no disabilities would normally receive a given treatment, then that treatment must be made available to anyone with disabilities who also has that medical problem. As a protection against discrimination in health care, the Americans with Disabilities Act has been important. Its commitments also lead to use of costly and weighty treatments in elderly persons with serious and progressive disabilities like dementia. Demented nursing-home patients sometimes have implanted defibrillators because they have no family or advance directive that could instruct providers to forego the treatment. The dementia patient who goes through defibrillator implantation in order to put off a peaceable natural death ordinarily gets to live through a more prolonged decline and, overall, a much more difficult dying. In my view, this has to be among the more incomprehensible practices that well-meaning policies have engendered. Yet it is not easy to see how to disassemble this legal structure without harming the fragile endeavor to ensure the rights and access to health care for people with disabilities (Gostin 2003).

Thus, the priorities in this arena might include

Reworking our language toward accurate descriptions of trade-offs for dementia patients among comfort, reliability, life extension, and peaceable dying

Building a public discourse about the nature and desirability of the variety of lives possible with severe dementia, so that a general consensus might emerge

Trying out strategies to limit use of high-cost but effective treatments in dementia patients

Shaping financing and regulation to allow trials of warranted reforms

FORCES THAT DISCOURAGE INNOVATION

Building a new and better care system tailored to long-term, eventually fatal chronic illness requires learning how to assess its strengths and weaknesses and how to arrange, finance, and regulate its services. That learning requires innovation, evaluation, and research. Some of this work is small-scale innovation that would usually be within the scope of approval by those managing programs or providing professional services: for example, trying out a new staffing pattern for nurses or a better way to ensure pain assessment and relief. Some of it involves broad social innovation, like changes in eligibility, coverage, or payment rates. Other parts of the work take the form of organized formal research, with control groups and defined interventions.

Society can take various actions to encourage or to discourage innovation. In the early years of the United States, public policies allowing people to leave bankruptcy behind and encouraging them to take risks on new investments helped engineer an era of invention and development. At present, substantial forces act to discourage innovation and encourage continuation of "accepted practices." Conventional liability litigation, for example, has been a strong force against change in health care generally, since there is often a period of heightened risk as a new approach takes root.

Increasingly, concern for the protection of human subjects complicates innovation as well. In order to ensure that human subjects of experimentation are knowledgeable about their risks (of harms and of loss of privacy) and that they consent freely, a set of rules and protections is in place, requiring substantial review of the research plan, the consent provisions, and the implementation of the research. The processes that govern research are weighty and often very slow (Lynn 2004; Casarett, Karlawish, and Sugarman 2000; Dubler and Bellin 2001).

Whether innovation, program redefinition, continuous quality improvement, and other reform endeavors count as research, and whether they should, is a subject of current concern (Lynn 2004; Lo and Groman

2003). If data-guided quality improvement must be regulated as research, the pace of change will be much slower than otherwise. If not, then society may need to articulate alternative arrangements in order to ensure that reformers treat patients equitably and with respect. In the absence of a clear process, the fears of liabilities and the demand to act conservatively could be major sources of delay and inaction.

Approaches to these problems might include

Limiting risks from liability litigation arising from thoughtful innovation

Building consensus on the boundaries of "research" for the purposes of reviewing plans for the protection of human subjects

Formulating responsible arrangements for protecting participants in innovation and reforms that are not "research"

Maintaining an impetus for innovation, learning, and rapid reforms

Avoiding Low-Impact Reforms

In a field that is so new and so complex, and in which the need for rapid improvements is becoming apparent, an array of possible reforms has come to the fore. Legalizing physician-assisted suicide is one idea that many states have considered. And as inflation and new treatment modalities create pressure on the income stream, nearly every provider group is adjusting its payment rates. Some advocates feel that revising the content of the education of physicians and nurses would improve the quality of care; others focus on making palliative care into a specialty parallel to cardiology or vascular surgery (Butler, Meier, and Nyberg 2003).

My guess is that these may all turn out to be low-leverage changes. Even if they all were accomplished, end-of-life care would not be greatly improved. Few patients want, and in good care fewer would want, suicide. Better payment rates for current providers won't change the incentives or dysfunctions. Teaching practitioners about good care may be essential, but it does not actually implement good care. And care delivery certainly needs more fundamental change than just adding a specialty. Of course, some of these reforms might actually have substantial adverse effects. Legalizing physician-assisted suicide might blunt our commitment to care for one another; and increasing payments or granting a protected status to certified specialists might encourage them to resist more fundamental change. Mainly, though, many of these issues would precipitate quite a struggle and demand energies that probably should be applied to other agendas.

In short, while it may well be important to pursue some of these issues some of the time, efficient reform depends in part upon forging and pursuing high-leverage strategies and avoiding spending much effort on low-leverage ones. Confidence about predictions of this sort is elusive. Nevertheless, since we have rarely even tried to strategize among the broad array of concerned parties, reformers in this arena could undoubtedly do better strategic planning, looking both for promising areas for major reforms and for areas of diminished importance. One major deficiency is that potential reformers do not now meet one another or work together, because we are split among diseases, specialties, settings of care, and vocational identities. Furthermore, we do not have galvanizing aims to share.

Some possibilities that might improve on the current uncoordinated efforts include

Convening key stakeholders and others experienced in reform efforts specifically to consider the possibilities for reforms and to gain accord on a list of priority agendas for all to pursue (Institute of Medicine 2004)

Organizing regional and statewide trials of major innovations (Institute of Medicine 2002)

The job of restructuring and refocusing care for the last part of life has to become a valued task. Professionals and civic leaders must see the undesirability of slowing it down with diversions or regulation and liabilities. Reformers need to establish a few venues for strategic planning that can generate loyalty and commitment among a broad array of advocates. Especially when moving from fee-for-service to a more flexible capitation or salary financing, society generally must make peace with the care system having some limits. It will not be possible to pay for all that we might want. Developing processes and trade-offs that the community supports will be challenging—and essential. The caregiver shortage and the dramatic dysfunctions in care present opportunities to build better care.

The Case for Reforming U.S. Health Care
Committee on Quality of Health Care in America,
Institute of Medicine

The American health care delivery system is in need of fundamental change. . . . Americans should be able to count on receiving care that meets their needs and is based on the best scientific knowledge. Yet there is strong evidence that this frequently is not the case. . . . Quality problems are everywhere, affecting many patients. Between the health care we have and the care we could have lies not just a gap, but a chasm.

The health care system as currently structured does not, as a whole, make the best use of its resources. . . . What is perhaps most disturbing is the absence of real progress toward restructuring health care systems to address both quality and cost concerns, or toward applying advances in information technology to improve administrative and clinical processes. . . . For several decades, the needs of the American public have been shifting from predominantly acute, episodic care to care for chronic conditions. Chronic conditions are now the leading cause of illness, disability, and death; they affect almost half of the U.S. population and account for the majority of health care expenditures.

The committee is confident that Americans can have a health care system of the quality they need, want, and deserve. But we are also confident that this higher level of quality cannot be achieved by further stressing current systems of care. The current care systems cannot do the job. Trying harder will not work. Changing systems of care will.

The committee proposes six aims for improvement to address key dimensions in which today's health care system functions at considerably lower levels than it can and should. Health care should be:

Safe . . .

Effective . . .

Patient-centered . . .

Timely . . .

Efficient . . .

Equitable . . .

The committee recognizes the enormity of the changes that will be required to achieve a substantial improvement in the nation's health care system. Although steps can be taken immediately to . . . redesign . . . health care, widespread application will require commitment to the provision of evidence-based care that is responsive to individual patients' needs and preferences. Well-designed and well-run systems of care will be required as well. These changes will occur most rapidly in an environment in which public policy and market forces are aligned and in which the change process is supported by an appropriate information technology infrastructure. . . .

. . . [C]are that is responsive to patient needs and makes consistent use of the best evidence requires far more conscious and careful organization than we find today.

Organizations will need to negotiate successfully six major challenges. The first is to redesign care processes to serve more effectively the needs of the chronically ill for coordinated, seamless care across settings and clinicians and over time. . . . A second challenge is making effective use of information technologies. . . . A third challenge is to manage the growing knowledge base and ensure that all those in the health care workforce have the skills they need. . . . A fourth challenge for organizations is coordination of care across patient conditions, services, and settings over time. . . . A fifth challenge is to continually advance the effectiveness of teams. . . . Finally, all organizations—whether or not health care related—can improve their performance only by incorporating care process and outcome measures into their daily work. Use of such measures makes it possible to understand the degree to which performance is consistent with best practices, and the extent to which patients are being helped. . . .

To enable the profound changes in health care recommended in this report, the *environment* of care must also change. . . . Two types of environmental change are needed:

· Focus and align the environment toward the six aims for improvement; and

· Provide, where possible, assets and encouragement for positive change.

The changes needed to realize a substantial improvement in health care involve the health care system as a whole. The new rules set forth in this report will affect the role, self-image, and work of front-line doctors, nurses, and other staff. . . .

American health care is beset by serious problems, but they are not intractable. Perfect care may be a long way off, but much better care is within our grasp. The committee envisions a system that uses the best knowledge, that is focused intensely on patients, and that works across health care providers and settings. . . . The committee believes that achieving such a system is both possible and necessary.

Adapted with permission from Institute of Medicine. 2001. *Crossing the quality chasm: a new health system for the twenty-first century.* Committee on Quality of Health Care in America, Institute of Medicine, ed. Washington, DC: National Academies Press, pp. 1–21.

5

GOOD CARE FOR US ALL

Building the Care System to Count On

Very sick people should not have to be afraid of their care system. They and their families need care they can count on, with the services that matter to them readily available. Since patients coming to the end of life ordinarily get care in various settings and from various providers—home care, doctor's office, hospice, hospital—the level of performance in each setting and from each provider must be high, and transfers among settings must be smooth. Only then can clinicians make promises of reliable services that cover all of the time from the onset of serious illness to the end of life. Meeting the important needs of patients and families when people face eventually fatal chronic conditions means

Developing a vision of good care that is worth achieving

Confronting entrenched and problematic barriers

Forging the will to make change happen

One way to envision the goal in care for the last part of life is to seek a set of care arrangements in which sick people do not need to be "lucky" in order to have the care and support they need, at the right time, every time. Within such a reliable system, patients, families, and loved ones can concentrate on living fully in the time left.

For Americans for Better Care of the Dying, an education and advocacy organization focused on the last part of life (www.abcd-caring.org), I articulated a vision of good care, embodied in a set of promises that doctors and nurses should be able to make, from early in the course of serious illness through to death.

Seven Promises Your Doctor Should Be Able to Make
- Evidence-based appropriate medical treatment
- Prevention and effective treatment of troubling symptoms
- Continuity, coordination, and comprehensiveness, so that essential services are in place when you need them
- Advance care planning so that common complications of your illness rarely create emergencies
- Customized care, reflecting your preferences and respecting your wishes
- Thoughtful use of the resources you and your family bring to bear (financial, emotional, and practical)
- Help that allows you to make the best of every day that you live

The key idea is not just a list of tasks enumerating what a care system should endeavor to deliver but insistence that delivery has to be reliable. Providers serving patients who live with fatal chronic illness today cannot promise these performance characteristics to patients, certainly not from the onset of illness all the way through to the end of life. Hospice programs can often deliver on these promises for the short time that patients are with them, and many "gem" programs manage to do a good job for a small number of patients or in a certain setting of care (see the examples in chapter 3). Patients might feel they're on a roulette wheel: things may work out fairly well or they may not, and it's nearly impossible to improve the odds.

These seven promises are substantially the same as a set of precepts of palliative care published by Last Acts (www.lastacts.org) and a set of guidelines for care at the end of life (American Geriatrics Society 1997). A care system that could make these seven promises would need to have these basic characteristics of clinical quality:

Excellent general medical skills, so that all interventions are in accord with evidence as to their likely merits, including medications, treatments, diagnostic issues, and prevention

Immediate on-call access (twenty-four hours a day, seven days a week) to a clinician who knows the patient and family and can always refer to the medical record, including the diagnoses, care plan, and advance planning directives

Extensive support and respect for family caregivers, including respite care, counseling, and training in needed home health tasks

Culturally and individually appropriate counseling about prognosis, treatment, advance care planning, and spiritual and emotional issues concerning the end of life

Reliable symptom prevention and relief (at least for pain, shortness of breath, depression, delirium, and skin breakdown)

A range of appropriate social and medical services, including interdisciplinary team care, medical and rehabilitation specialists, financial planning, and personal care when needed

These are not terribly costly interventions, though making them reliable will entail some added costs. Perhaps we could learn to forego some costly treatments that carry only small benefits, which probably would allow good care to be no more costly than current dysfunctional patterns of care. Whatever balance of costs and painful decisions about costs that society achieves, it is certainly the case that excellent care has to be sustainable: that is, within society's ability to generate funds, human resources, and living arrangements.

Furthermore, the style and method for high-quality care systems will have to emphasize professionalism, caring, efficiency, and an ongoing search for new insights and patterns that ensure continued improvement. Certainly, we do not know enough today to design the optimally achievable care system for twenty years from now. Only by vigorously seeking to learn what we need to learn can we hope to generate reliable care delivery arrangements in the twenty years before the baby boomers start to need care for serious chronic illness.

One area of special focus must be the development of supportive arrangements for paid and unpaid caregivers. Improvements will depend upon these human resources, so optimal care arrangements must include some combination of improved benefits, pay, respect, career ladders, and emotional support for caregivers. At least through 2030, the country will have to keep developing additional capacity to serve the onslaught of boomers coming to their last years of life.

Reliable care at an affordable price for people living with fatal chronic illness is possible, but to achieve it we need insight, innovation, and commitment. Reform would build on Medicare, which enjoys wide support as a social commitment to the elderly, and on other programs that use public funds to provide broad access to medical services. We know how to arrange good care, and many of the improved approaches are either cost-neutral or of modest cost. Furthermore, rather than meekly accepting the system's shortcomings, the baby-boom generation is likely—first as caregivers, and then as aging and dying people—to rally political support for more reliable care.

Reprise of the Current Situation

American health care builds on the assumptions that the physician and the hospital are the central service elements, that short bursts of services define the course, and that categories that define care plans mostly depend on diagnosis. Quality issues revolve around performance of definitive interventions, such as operations or procedures, or focus on preventive services, such as early treatment of hypertension or childhood immunization. While these strategies meet the care needs of generally healthy people and those who have minor or curable ailments, these patterns and assumptions do not meet the needs of people with severe and eventually fatal illness (see figure 5, in chapter 2). In fact, the way that our culture defines good care actually creates barriers to reform, because it does not name or measure shortcomings in the last phase of life. When we take the Web site of Nursing Home Compare (www.cfmc.org/nhqi/nhprqi_compare.htm) or accreditation by the Joint Commission on Accreditation of Healthcare Organizations (www.jcaho.org/htba/index.htm) or record reviews from the National Committee on Quality Assurance's Health Plan Employer Data and Information Set (www.ncqa.org/programs/HEDIS) to be authoritative standards of quality care, we may forget that they measure very little of importance to a person facing fatal chronic illness.

Continuity of the care plan and care team across time and sites is essential for patients who will be ill and disabled for the remainder of their lives. Yet physician and hospital care for those with eventually fatal chronic illness is mostly tied to episodes of acute worsening, and few professionals stay central to the care for the duration of patients' lives. Severely ill patients often see an array of specialists, typically in the office or hospital, though they may also receive many supportive services at home or in nursing facilities. Their doctors are usually only dimly aware of the nonmedical services or the patients' and families' way of life. Patients may be referred from one physician to another, or transferred from one setting to another, without the benefit of a common understanding of their situation or even a common medical record accessible to each provider. An error in diagnosing an abscess would be criticized and addressed. But shortcomings that arise from lost advance care plans (precipitating a futile or unwanted attempt at resuscitation or an unnecessary transfer from nursing home to hospital) or delays in important medications or tests are rarely seen as outrageous—or even as medical errors—but are accepted as simply part of how the work gets done (Loxtercamp 1996; Lynn, Harrold, and Ayers 1997; Myers and Lynn 2002; Lynn and Goldstein 2003).

Indeed, many providers never learn of the problems that result from shortcomings in care planning and coordination. Physicians who see a patient in the hospital often do not expect to see or hear about that patient again. But if they knew about a problem—such as the patient's lack of a plan for turning off an implanted defibrillator as his Parkinson's disease worsens, or the patient's difficulties in getting prescribed opioids delivered to her home in a poor part of the city—they might be able to plan ahead and avoid it. The current system is set up at best for short-term goals: discharge alive or error-free medication administration. The academic physician who sees patients for one month each year and spends the rest of the year in research is not expected to follow up on the patients' progress, nor is the "doc in the box" at an acute-care drop-in center or emergency room. Hospitals have no financial incentive and little legal responsibility to be concerned about the performance of a patient's care providers beyond discharge—so no one faults them for being shortsighted. Even the current researchers and commentators on error prevention and patient safety have not addressed how to deal with errors that later providers notice when they receive patients after a few transfers.

These problems are receiving sustained attention in a remarkable program of reports by the Institute of Medicine. Their most visible products to date are *Crossing the Quality Chasm: A New Health System for the Twenty-First Century* (2001) and *To Err Is Human: Building a Safer Health Care System* (1999b). These scholarly reports show that our care system is seriously unsafe and generally dysfunctional and that many of its shortcomings arise from not having adapted to the realities of chronic illness and its needs. The *Chasm* report puts forth the claim that good care needs to be safe, effective, efficient, personalized, timely, and equitable. (See excerpt, pp. 118–20.) It also outlines a vision of how to achieve those ends. Much of this book applies that vision to the neediest people, those sick enough to die.

Too often, health-care providers do not plan for—or acknowledge—the fact that patients are seriously ill and will never again be well. Advance care planning (Hammes and Rooney 1998; Hammes 2001) is not widely or consistently done. As a result, many patients miss a valuable opportunity to plan for the kinds of risks and experiences that their situation entails or for the kinds of responses they would prefer. Given the opportunity, people could make the various arrangements that would increase the likelihood of living as they wished in whatever time they have left. Because most people with chronic diseases have an unpredictable course to death, the failure to begin advance planning early in the course of the disease can lead to hasty decisions made while in distress or providing treatment "on autopilot," rather than decisions shaped by each patient's possibilities and preferences.

Gradually, this situation is improving. In Oregon now, most nursing-home residents and home-care recipients have a written plan, called the Physician Orders for Life-Sustaining Treatments (POLST), that directs important aspects of care in an emergency (Americans for Better Care of the Dying 1999). The Veterans Health Care System made advance care planning for veterans with serious illnesses a priority and part of the formula for leadership funds, strategies that got plans made for most of their seriously ill patients within a year (Americans for Better Care of the Dying 2001). Clearly, care delivery systems can improve advance care planning.

Physicians and other health-care providers often learn very little about serious disability and the potential to improve function and relieve or prevent pain and suffering (Billings and Block 1997; Institute of Medicine 1997). This material is nearly nonexistent in medical school curricula and in medical and other health-care textbooks (Rabow et al. 2000; Carron, Lynn, and Keaney 1999; Callahan 1995; Ferrell et al. 2000). However, several groundbreaking programs are working to remedy this lack of training, including the Education for Physicians on End-of-Life Care (EPEC) Project (2001), from the American Medical Association; the End-of-Life Nursing Education Consortium (ELNEC) (2000), from the American Association of Colleges of Nursing; and the End of Life/Palliative Education Resource Center (EPERC) (2001). Some states have mandated at least a small amount of continuing education so that current practitioners might catch up with essential knowledge (State Medical Licensure Requirements and Statistics 2003).

In sum, the deficiencies are striking, but a number of elements are in place to make substantial and sustainable reforms possible.

Trajectories Form a Basis for Achievable Excellence

Use of the three illness trajectories (described in chapter 2) as a framework simplifies and organizes the task of tailoring services to fit the patient population. The next sections characterize the priority elements of clinical services for persons living through each trajectory and give sample cases illuminating the contrast between current patterns and what could be the standard of excellent care.

SHORT PERIOD OF EVIDENT DECLINE — TYPICAL OF CANCER

Case Study

A common current scenario

The Main Street Church support group for advanced cancer patients meets every week, and this week, like many others, the conversation turns to the reality and the fear of pain. AB has a doctor who would not give anything very strong yet, "because you'll need those strong drugs later." Only when she got her granddaughter, a nurse, to help her change doctors did she get comfortable enough even to come to the support group meetings. CD had a problem getting a pharmacy to fill his prescription, and none would deliver it to his part of town: "Too dangerous." EF had just come home from the hospital where he had been in terrible pain for days while the house staff and attending physician made adjustments in his medications on morning rounds each day. It took a week before he got comfortable enough to sleep or eat. GH was not at the meeting, being "too exhausted from not sleeping," since she moved into a nursing home, because she could not take her medications when she wanted them. The social worker coordinating the support group helped participants deal with their anger and frustration. However, a family member pointed out that "you can't get mad at the doctor or you'll never get anything done."

Achievable excellence

The Main Street Church support group for advanced cancer patients meets every week, and usually the topic is about family concerns and spiritual issues. AB mentioned that her mother was scared that AB would be left miserable when she went to the local university hospital for a special treatment, because her aunt had had that experience ten years ago. Her mother was delighted to find that things had changed and the care was excellent, right down to asking about comfort and ensuring it. CD reflected on the conversation with his doctor about his fears that pain might "get out of hand" as his cancer got worse, but his doctor was able to reassure him that pain would never be overwhelming, using data from the regional cancer alliance interviews with patients and family members about their experiences. EF and GH moved the conversation along to other topics, because there is just not much to say about pain when everyone is confident that it will never be allowed to be overwhelming.

Adapted with permission from Institute of Medicine. 2003. *Priority areas for national action: transforming health care quality.* Committee on Identifying Priority Areas for Quality Improvement, Institute of Medicine. Adams K, Corrigan J, eds. Washington, DC: National Academies Press, p. 82.

A highly reliable care system for the usual cancer trajectory would:

Build ongoing advance care planning into early treatment, modifying the plan as the disease progresses

Provide prevention and treatment for symptoms and rehabilitation for disabilities throughout the course of illness

Provide some costly "aggressive" treatments even very late in the illness, because they still work to enhance the patient's life

Smooth the transition from office-based care to care at home (mostly hospice care) as the patient becomes more ill

Attend to family needs and spiritual/emotional issues throughout

How could we organize to accomplish these ends? In this case, hospice is a natural answer. The weeks to months of dramatic losses in function, weight, and comfort call for the interdisciplinary teams, continuity, family support, and preparations for death that mark hospice. Integration of hospice with comprehensive cancer care (see the case study describing the Ireland Cancer Center, in chapter 3) would get these services started early enough to support patients and families throughout the course. The key providers would probably be oncologists, cancer centers, and hospice programs, with additional support from nursing homes, home-care providers, and assisted-living facilities. Perhaps comprehensive cancer centers and hospice programs could take responsibility for ensuring that hospice care at home and in nursing homes is reliably available, of good quality, and regularly used with smooth, error-free transfers.

CHRONIC ILLNESS WITH EXACERBATIONS AND SUDDEN DYING — TYPICAL OF ORGAN SYSTEM FAILURE

Case Study

A common current scenario

Mr. CV lived with his wife in a small duplex, and their son lived nearby. As Mr. CV became more disabled with heart attacks and progressive heart failure, his living arrangements became more constrained. They moved his bed to the living room, built a long ramp to the door, and changed the family diet to avoid salt. Nevertheless, he would go into an episode of "failure" every few months and would be rushed to the hospital by the emergency ambulance, struggling to breathe. His wife lived in terror of these episodes and just shook and trembled for days afterward. She had lived through breast cancer and a stroke herself, and she worried all the time about what would happen to him if she died first, and what would happen to her if he died first! Their assets had been spent, and they routinely skimped on their prescription medications, since otherwise they could not meet the rent and food bills. Their son helped out by keeping the place repaired, but he worked as a clerk in a convenience store and did not really have funds to help.

Every time Mr. CV was hospitalized, he had a different set of doctors. They never even seemed to have the medical record. Between hospitalizations, he was scheduled for a follow-up visit in "resident's clinic," but he did not usu-

ally go, since it cost so much to get the taxis and seemed to do very little good. He did not understand his medications, did not weigh himself, did not know what to do if he was starting to get short of breath, and did not have any conversations with any physicians that implied that this condition would eventually take his life.

Achievable excellence

Mr. CV and his wife were enrolled in a complex care-management program that ensured that they had good medical services and help with financial planning, family support, and advance care planning. They both came to understand how to manage medicines and weight, and what extra medications to take at the earliest signs of trouble. He had only two more hospitalizations, one for prostate trouble and one for heart failure brought on by a bad cold with a fever. As his condition worsened, nurses also came to see him at home. As planned, he died at home, and the same care team continued to support his wife with the health and living challenges she faced.

Adapted with permission from Institute of Medicine. 2003. *Priority areas for national action: transforming health care quality.* Committee on Identifying Priority Areas for Quality Improvement, Institute of Medicine. Adams K, Corrigan J, eds. Washington, DC: National Academies Press, p. 63.

A highly reliable care system for the person with an advanced chronic organ system failure trajectory would focus first on:

Teaching patients and families the essentials of disease management, primarily how to recognize symptoms and prevent worsening of illness

Ensuring constant availability of key medications

Planning and making decisions about treatments in the event of a sudden severe exacerbation

Providing early intervention (over the telephone or in person at home) for the earliest signs of exacerbation

Offering in-home adaptations and equipment (for example, oxygen) to ensure patients' comfort

Tailoring the care plan to patients and their families

Providing care at home, if preferred, for the end of life

In good care for advanced organ system failure, prevention and early treatment of exacerbations alleviate suffering, reduce costs, and delay death. The major service providers would be nurses with advanced training who are familiar with the medications and physiology and who can call on other professionals from an interdisciplinary team as needed, such as medical specialists, social workers, pastoral counselors, and occupational therapists. When patients want to forego or stop aggressive life support, aggressive symptom relief must be reliably available (National Coalition for Health Care and Institute for Healthcare Improvement 2000; Brumley, Enguidanos, and Cherin 2003; Lynn, Schall, et al. 2000; Lynn and Goldstein 2003; Quill and Byock 2000).

A LONG DWINDLING—
TYPICAL OF FRAILTY AND DEMENTIA

Case Study

A common current scenario

KL, now eighty-nine, has had a rough few years. Her son would say it all started with a fall at home, which broke her hip. She has never been "able to manage things" since the surgery on her hip. She had to give up her little house and move in with her son and daughter-in-law. Even so, she could not get around when they were out and spent many days just sitting in bed or in a chair. She actually had been having memory problems before the fall, and now she cannot remember her family or her name, though she is still able to feed herself. She is incontinent but won't wear diapers, so the family does a lot of laundry. Every few months, something seems to go awry and she ends up in the hospital—for pneumonia, bowel blockage, confusion, or whatever. Each time she comes home, KL has a new set of medications and problems. Last time it was a pressure sore over her tailbone from sitting on a bedpan too long. Her son and his wife, now old enough for Medicare themselves, are weary of the physical labor involved in her care and feel their own health and life slipping away. Yet they don't want to send her to the Medicaid-accepting nursing home, which is miles away from them and anyone else she knows. Her doctors see KL in their offices, trips that require all-day efforts from the family. She has some home health visits occasionally for one thing or another, but none are regular enough to feel like reliable help, and none attend to the family's concerns or issues of environmental safety. She has no advance care plans, not even a decision between her son and her doctor about whether she should undergo resuscitation.

Achievable excellence

The doctor and elder-care nurse noticed that KL and her family needed some extra attention a few years ago, when she first came to clinic bruised from falling in her garden. Since then, she has mostly had doctor visits at home, even having her blood drawn and her X-rays taken there. She did make a planned move from her little home into the shelter of her son's home, but they get regular respite care so that family members can attend to their own needs and take trips. Her mind is failing, but the physical arrangements have been modified to keep her safe and to make her care easier on the family. She got the bathroom bars and bedside commode she needed right away, the home environment is as safe as possible, and a call-in device functions as an alarm to summon help. She and her family made plans early as to how she should live out the end of life. Those plans include a decision not to have 911 transport to the hospital, but to have an in-home emergency geriatrics team come for any urgent situation. They agreed on no resuscitation. Indeed, before she became too confused to do so, she even picked out the hymns she wants to have sung at her funeral and made arrangements for all the details she could. She is comfortable. Her family is doing a lot of work, but everyone says it is fairly meaningful and important, and all expect her to live this way until a major complication arises and leads to death.

The dementia and frailty trajectory requires further adaptation of the service array. For these patients, a primary focus must be on supporting family caregivers and providing concrete services on an everyday basis.

Day-care centers, home health aides, Meals on Wheels, legal aid, family respite, behavioral management, and nursing homes are at the heart of the service array. While cancer patients might be very sick for a year, and organ system failure patients could be sick, off and on, for a few years, dementia and frailty patients can often live for a decade with increasing symptoms and increasing disability. Thus, the care system must accommodate very long durations of progressive illness and adapt to changing family situations, slow decline in the patients' capabilities, and either a sudden or lingering death.

MediCaring: From Promises to Practical Program

The care system we now have reflects its origins—powerful men who were worried about heart attacks. That is an outrageous oversimplification, of course, but still fundamentally true. A citizen can get 911 services almost anywhere in the country; and surgeries, devices, drugs, and hospitals have had ongoing investment and yield profits. But don't risk finding that you need a home health aide on the weekend or need help opening a jar on the day your arthritis acts up! "We don't DO that" is the likely answer. The hopes and fears of elderly ladies living in walk-up apartments and juggling half a dozen medical problems along with small incomes and rising rents are quite different from the issues that built the care system. For all those elderly women (and a fair number of frail old men, too), endurance and constancy count for a lot, as do concrete services in daily life and respect for the human value of home, control, companionship, and meaningfulness. The emergency squad that rescues the heart attack victim on the subway platform, the hospital that gets him to surgery within a few hours, and the pharmaceutical suppliers that help keep this from happening again can reasonably be concerned just with fixing his problem and walking away. The social service agency trying to keep an elderly, mildly memory-impaired, and impoverished lady at home and comfortable does not really have a problem to fix. Instead, it is trying to avert calamity, to ensure safety, and simply to help her keep

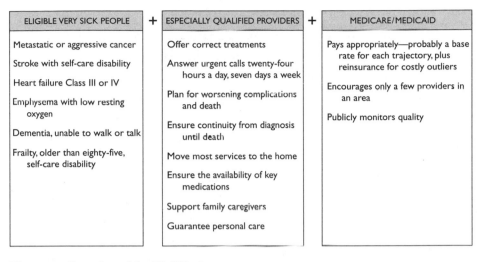

ELIGIBLE VERY SICK PEOPLE	+	ESPECIALLY QUALIFIED PROVIDERS	+	MEDICARE/MEDICAID
Metastatic or aggressive cancer		Offer correct treatments		Pays appropriately—probably a base rate for each trajectory, plus reinsurance for costly outliers
Stroke with self-care disability		Answer urgent calls twenty-four hours a day, seven days a week		
Heart failure Class III or IV				Encourages only a few providers in an area
Emphysema with low resting oxygen		Plan for worsening complications and death		Publicly monitors quality
Dementia, unable to walk or talk		Ensure continuity from diagnosis until death		
Frailty, older than eighty-five, self-care disability		Move most services to the home		
		Ensure the availability of key medications		
		Support family caregivers		
		Guarantee personal care		

Figure 7. Overview of the MediCaring strategy.

herself clean, fed, and engaged as long as possible. These services do not attract investment—their funding is usually a welfare or safety-net model of the least expense possible without scandal. The care system the elderly lady needs would have very different priorities and structures. Current care arrangements simply expect her to use the system that other priorities generated.

Various clinical service providers around the country are working with a mental model of optimum care, sometimes called MediCaring (a term trademarked by Americans for Better Care of the Dying), which aims for more effective organization of care services (see figure 7). Basically, the core idea is that we could identify a time near the onset of substantial disability and suffering from progressive, eventually fatal chronic illness and, starting then, match the patient to a tailored service array with appropriate funding and regulation. For each of the three major trajectories, eligibility would be set by the onset of a specific serious level of the patient's condition. For example, for persons facing mostly heart failure problems, eligibility might be determined by an inability to climb steps because of shortness of breath and having the heart move less than 30 percent of its volume on each stroke. The actual eligibility criteria mainly need to be replicable and administratively feasible rather than comporting with a predetermined physiological standard. In general, they would reflect the results of the "no surprise" question: people sick enough that it would be no surprise if they died within the coming year. Services would be tailored to ensure continuity, advance care planning, family support, and other important elements.

This approach offers the opportunity to blend the interdisciplinary team, continuity, and symptom relief that underlie the effectiveness of hospice with the self-care education, timely reminders for prevention, and advance care planning of successful chronic illness management. The most sensible funding plan would be based mostly on capitation or on a budget, probably with separate coverage of occasional costly "outliers" like heart transplants. MediCaring is the kind of major rethinking of health-care delivery that offers hope of substantial reform, especially since the providers would have to meet quality standards in order to be eligible for the increased payments. Not only are there a dozen providers trying out this set of ideas, in settings from veterans' home care to hospice, but the Medicare Payment Advisory Commission (2003) has declared that it will examine whether disease management programs might target beneficiaries coming to the end of life. Similar trial programs are included in the legislation that enables Medicare to cover prescription drugs (Medicare Prescription Drug, Improvement, and Modernization Act 2003).

The deficiencies that now plague heart failure care (see chapter 4) might make it an especially appealing case study for early implementation of a MediCaring approach. If Medicare provided enhanced payment for care of persons with advanced heart failure, perhaps as a management fee or a comprehensive payment (like PACE or hospice), then Medicare might also require that providers demonstrate certain performance characteristics in order to qualify for that payment. For example, the provider team might be required to guarantee that an appropriate clinician could be at the home within two hours, day or night; to make plans for exacerbations with essentially all patients; to provide care in hospital and nursing home as well as home care and office visits; and to ensure self-care education and family support. Since heart failure affects many people covered by Medicare and since better care patterns are well proven by research but only rarely available, this might be an area in which reforms could start. Working with heart failure would teach us how to allow programs to reach a sustainable size, how to reinsure for costly outliers, how to curtail routine use of high-cost treatments of dubious value, and how to advocate for sustained reforms.

MediCaring programs for heart failure turn out to be closely linked to similar work for lung failure. Thus, fielding good care arrangements could effectively cover most patients who follow the second trajectory—chronic organ system failure. Traditional hospice programs caring for cancer patients provide the model for the cancer trajectory. That would leave us to struggle with frailty and dementia, the third trajectory. The split in resources between Medicare, Medicaid, and private assets complicates handling the course for these patients and families. Demonstration programs might build upon PACE (see chapter 3), for example, by exploring the possibilities of actuarial pay-outs from private wealth in order to enter a care system that is reliable and comprehensive.

The basic ideas in MediCaring are these:

To reform payment policy and clinical services nearly simultaneously

To provide clinical services that match the care needs as sorted by trajectory, especially the requirements for continuity, services at the home or nursing home, caregiver support, and advance care planning

To pay at an appropriate rate and with enough flexibility so that programs can manage a broad range of varying patients without recourse to special funding supplements

To require nearly all provider arrangements to last through all of serious illness until death (and bereavement)

Thereby to create a structure that can balance the merits of interventions and work within sustainable resource constraints

This proposal is rather different from those that add a layer of useful coordination to the underlying care system, such as disease management; and it is rather different from just paying for usual care at a discounted risk-adjusted rate. Improvements in payment policy should generally link to high-value care, so that only providers capable of effective and efficient care can sustain their business model. That is what MediCaring aims to do.

Methods to Achieve Reform

Evidence from other areas of health care suggests that sweeping change is possible if we give high enough priority to the problem at hand. For example, up to a few decades ago, childbirth practices were decidedly inadequate, and new mothers used to be "lucky" if their experience with childbirth was relatively comfortable and free of complications. Now childbirth has become routinely safer, and parents are quite involved in planning for labor and delivery. Just as new mothers who experienced comfortable, complication-free births were considered "lucky" in years past, Americans feel "lucky" today if a loved one has a relatively comfortable experience with a serious chronic disease and ensuing death. Also, just as childbirth protocols came to value human aspects of the childbirth experience, so might protocols and practices evolve to guide care for serious chronic illness at the end of life. Of course, each situation presents its own unique challenges and opportunities, and the parallel with obstetrics breaks down at various points. Nevertheless, study of the methods of change used in reforming other social practices and health care might well provide insights into how to engineer reforms for this population.

Certainly, no method is more important than innovation with evaluation (Kendall et al. 2003). We need a few years of trying out promising ideas and learning which ones actually serve us well. A recent publication by an Institute of Medicine committee recommends various demonstration projects for Medicare (Institute of Medicine 2003). The committee asks for one year of planning, three years of implementation, and an ensuing time for review and analysis. Though its approach gives reasonably reliable evaluation of the projects at issue, the method does not reflect their urgency. And more effective and dynamic strategies are readily available. Rather than test a settled intervention for three years, a steering committee could use ongoing feedback to reshape the intervention every few months. This approach, called rapid-cycle quality improvement, tests multiple elements in quick succession. It makes a remarkable engine of improvement for care in the last part of life (www.ihi.org; Lynn, Schuster, and Kabcenell 2000).

An old aphorism among reformers is that "you can't improve what you don't measure." Certainly, most successful projects to improve the public's health need to monitor trends, using population-based measurement. Yet we have no way to monitor what happens in populations at the end of life. Quite simply, no one knows the rates of serious pain, family bankruptcy, or advance care planning. No political leader can know whether things are improving or falling apart in his or her jurisdiction. But a few projects begin to shed light on the issues. For example, a research team in Oregon is tallying the experience of decedents through interviews with family members (Oregon Health Sciences University 2002). Last Acts recently published a report card on performance state by state (Last Acts 2002). Working out an epidemiology that would allow comparisons between locales and monitoring of trends would create a powerful tool to motivate the will for change and guide implementation (Singer and Wolfson 2003).

Living for a long time with fatal illness is still a new cultural phenomenon, and we have much to learn about how to make this time of life comfortable and rewarding for patients and families. Fortunately, good care does not have to await development of new drugs or devices. Medicine and nursing possess the tools to ensure comfort and dignity throughout the course of serious disease and dying, but their use is not efficiently built into care delivery. Reformers need the evidence from innovations to guide better strategies for care-system engineering.

The following questions are especially relevant to research, continuous quality improvement, and reflection:

Can severity and trajectory of a patient's condition serve as the criteria of eligibility for a set of care arrangements (discernibly different from those in the usual care system) that would stay in place through the rest of his or her life?

Would some small and feasible number of service arrays (like the three trajectories) provide well-adapted services to almost all persons living through eventually fatal chronic disease?

Do many people actually recover or move to another trajectory after qualifying for MediCaring in one trajectory?

Can we estimate the costs and insurance considerations (such as reinsuring high-cost outliers, numbers needed for predictable costs) for each trajectory?

Should reforms address a broad understanding of patients' and families' needs that includes housing and spiritual issues, or should they focus on conventionally "medical" issues?

Can we devise methods of payment for dually eligible persons (enrolled in Medicare and Medicaid, such as PACE) that account for private wealth and still yield coherent payment throughout fatal illness (such as reverse mortgages, prepurchase of packages of services like long-term care insurance or prepaid life care)?

Can we generate and tolerate social structures to constrain the use of very high-cost but effective treatments (like high-cost medications, implantable defibrillators, and dialysis) for patients in these trajectories?

Can we implement an epidemiology of the last years of life to monitor this population?

Can we hold public officials and professional leadership accountable for adverse trends identified by monitoring the epidemiology?

Can a broad array of providers and funders generate innovations and evaluations of alternative strategies for organizing and delivering care?

To answer these questions, we need to synthesize all our available data and experience into useful formats and action agendas. This work requires substantial investment, emotionally and financially, in a multiyear plan to build the knowledge and insight for a trustworthy care system.

Americans continue to wrestle with how to talk about and even how to imagine many aspects of life with long-term and severe disease, disability, and suffering. Few have yet come to terms with the increasingly likely prospect of long-term disability in the years near death; of coexisting and competing causes of death and suffering, which make eradication of a particular condition of only limited importance; and of prognosis as an inescapably ambiguous characteristic until very late in the course of fatal illness. Presumably, we can accelerate our awareness of people's needs toward the end of life and the ability of the community to meet those needs. We need to build a cultural store of traditions, stories, rituals, and meanings about the last phase of life; and we need to build that part of our culture as quickly as possible.

Leaders of a variety of allied fields—aging, health care, disability rights, public health, and medicine, for example—will need to find the mental models and the language that gradually reflect and sometimes create more accurate and useful ways to frame the issues. Rather than aiming to prevent death in the elderly, we may acknowledge that we will try to delay it. In place of a single cause of death, we will acknowledge multiple contributing causes; and in place of using the category of "dying," we will come to call it the last chapter or phase of life.

Working with the perspective of a span of survival might be more productive than working with age per se. The way to achieve reforms in culture and language may depend heavily on changes in news media and popular entertainment. The Last Acts Writers Project, which provides story ideas and vignettes to film and television screenwriters, thereby encourages them to include more realistic portrayals of living with serious illness and the end of life.

What should count as good—or as outrageous—quality of care for those with severe disabilities and suffering with eventually fatal chronic illness? Where are the standards of care for these populations? Just as national groups insist that good care include certain drugs after heart attacks and certain immunizations for adults, strong standards should direct the basics in end-of-life care. And as we once learned to reject racial segregation and to address domestic abuse, we need to become intolerant of the persistence of demonstrably inadequate care for those living with fatal chronic illness. Professionals and organizations should endorse standards of care like those listed here, even though only a minority of patients get this care at this time:

Care plans for most serious complications should be in place and readily available at all times for people with progressive and fatal chronic illness.

Pain and other symptoms should be prevented when possible and treated immediately when present.

If people find human presence comforting during the last phase of life, they should have company.

Families should be able to reach a clinician who knows them personally when they are frightened by a change in the patient's status at home.

An example of how errors in routine practice came to be viewed as just that—errors—comes from Oregon, which has enjoyed remarkable success with its Physician Orders for Life-Sustaining Treatment (Lynn,

Schuster, and Kabcenell 2000; Oregon Health Sciences University 2002;
Dunn et al. 1996). In one study, 180 nursing-home patients who had a
POLST and who were later admitted to hospitals did not receive CPR
and were not put on ventilators (Tolle et al. 1998). This excellent system
did not work in the case of an elderly woman admitted to an Oregon
Health Sciences University (OHSU) hospital. Although she had a
POLST on record at the nursing home where she was a resident, it did
not come with her when she came to the hospital in an emergency. Consequently, when the patient collapsed, she was put on a ventilator and received the usual array of life support. She died after a stay in the intensive-
care unit. However, not having the POLST upset hospital staff, who
viewed this case as a serious medical error. Staff filed reports, questioned
participants, and assessed root causes. As a result, administrators used the
case to examine a problem in the system and design ways to prevent it
from happening again (Americans for Better Care of the Dying 1999).

That sort of standard setting around the needs and priorities of this
population will have to happen many times, as the public and the professionals come to see what matters and how to achieve it reliably. So I do
believe that the care system at work in the United States within twenty
years will look very different from today's dominant models, but I also believe that we will get to that future with a long series of what seem to be
small changes. If reforms draw on innovations and evidence and are
backed by strong political forces, we can make improvements quickly.

Reforms to Implement Right Away!

How could we start the process of reform? I think rapid reform depends on
pursuing an array of attention-getting small endeavors that could create a
movement and investing in important longer-term efforts to build the evidence and shape the agenda. All of these activities would focus around creating a political force, broad clinical capability, and sustainable financing.

Short-term consciousness-raising is urgently needed and readily available, for example:

- Medicare should propose to pay half of a patient's second hospital-ization for the same serious chronic disease within a year, if the first hospitalization did not include any advance care planning. Just getting Medicare leadership to discuss this idea would probably trigger its salutary effects.

- Medicare should pay a 20 percent differential to the advantage of physicians who regularly provide continuity care for patients with serious chronic illness. This could be part of the current interest in "paying for performance."

- Public policies could start supporting family and paid caregivers—give them respite care, financial support, and health insurance. Again, just forcing the discussion into the public arena might gal-vanize support.

- Family caregivers should have a radio show, input into political campaigns, and organizations advocating for their issues.

- Medicare should initiate a set of demonstration projects that target those sick enough to die.

Building the evidence that can shape reform so that changes actually move health care toward efficient and effective strategies will require some longer-term perspectives:

- Direct the Centers for Disease Control and Prevention and the National Institute on Aging to develop an epidemiology of the last part of life and then to map trends over time and variations across jurisdictions.

- Direct research at the National Institutes of Health toward relief and prevention of symptoms.

- Test out the effects of alternative strategies for income support, in-centive alignment, and community control in services for serious chronic illness.

- Test out innovations in organizing nursing and clinical services.

Some of these require congressional action, leadership in federal executive agencies, or innovation by organized health-care delivery systems. Of course, if there were strong incentive to have those parties paying attention and addressing issues, we would already be moving along much more adeptly. Making small changes does matter, not only for improving care but also for forming the political will to make more substantial and enduring changes.

Forging the Will to Make Improvements Happen

For nearly every provider, payer, and patient, doing whatever was done yesterday is easier than doing something new, even if people expect the innovation to be an improvement. The strongest threat to substantial reform, over and over, is the persistent acceptability of the status quo. These are our "usual suspects" of habit, inertia, and inattention. Change is not likely without leaders able to articulate the need for a better approach, to envision what can be accomplished, and to encourage intolerance of current arrangements. Overcoming inertia requires a sense of urgency, outrage, or commitment.

A vision of better care comprises a reliable set of services that allow people in the last phase of life to live comfortably and meaningfully and give their families confidence about what is being done. Having care arrangements that enable patients to trust that the right services will be available at the right time is the important hallmark. Clinicians must be able to make those seven promises listed at the beginning of this chapter. The care system must demonstrably create desirable experiences such as comfort, confidence, life closure, and caregiver support and do this at a price that the community can afford. A final critical element is that the care arrangements must continue to adapt and evolve through ongoing learning and reassessment.

What might generate the will to achieve that vision? Here are some promising approaches:

· Publicize shortcomings in current care using epidemiology (over time and across populations) (Last Acts 2002) and through popular narratives such as news stories, television shows, or movies as well as scholarly reports (Institute of Medicine 2001).

· Also publicize examples of better care, such as "gem" programs that are doing something particularly well (American Hospital Association 2002; National Coalition for Health Care and Institute for Healthcare Improvement 2000 and 2002); evaluate innovations; and publish promising results widely, finding well-known spokespersons to disseminate the message.

· Expand the language and images about serious chronic illnesses and dying to highlight the shared needs of dying people and the shared concerns of caregivers, since identification wih a group provides the opportunity for political influence.

· Label shortcomings as outrages—call them "errors," "harms," "unprofessional conduct," or even "abuse."

· Convert key issues into political issues—reforming Medicare to serve this population and its family caregivers seems an obvious issue to include in political platforms.

· Illustrate to those who lead Medicaid programs, including governors and state directors, how Medicaid recipients living through the last part of life both receive inadequate services and run up large bills, and show that good care at a sustainable cost depends upon substantial reorganization.

· Engender a real sense of urgency by fostering a broad recognition of the burgeoning size of the affected population and the coming shortage of paid and informal caregivers.

· Encourage enlightened self-interest: the care system we build will be what we have for help when each of us cares for loved ones coming to the end of life and again when we ourselves get sick and die.

· Gain broad commitment to a shared agenda from professional associations, public interest advocates, political parties, and organizations focused upon particular problems (like pain), populations (the aging), or diseases (such as cancer or lung disease).

Highly visible people must articulate the will to change in order for change to be tolerated. Dr. Don Berwick gave a galvanizing talk in 1999 to the American College of Physicians–American Society of Internal Medicine, calling for these professionals to adopt this issue and provide leadership (Berwick 1999), but the follow-through foundered. Elected and appointed federal officials, including the president, the surgeon general, and the secretary of Health and Human Services, have not embraced this issue, either in the current administration or in previous ones. However, demographics ensure that the time is at hand. The announcement by the American Association of Retired Persons of its ten-year commitment to long-term care, chronic disease care, and end-of-life care may well be the sort of endeavor that builds the framework of reform. In December 2003, the Agency for Healthcare Research and Quality published the first congressionally mandated *National Healthcare Quality Report*, listing the four components of patient needs as staying healthy, getting better, living with illness or disability, and coping with the end of life (Agency for Healthcare Research and Quality 2003, 12). The obvious dearth of available information to include in the report on care for serious illness and disability and for the end of life might serve to goad funders and researchers to attend to the deficiencies.

Finally, of course, someone must actually do the work of building the better care system. As the knowledge base deepens and the will to move forward coalesces, we can expect at least incremental changes. Sometimes change will be sweeping, but often reforms can survive the political process only if they are perceived as small adjustments. Change always engenders opposition, at least from those comfortable with the current situation. As providers come to understand that building a system for fatal chronic illness probably means a much smaller proportion of the available income for some traditional anchors of health care, and much less power as well, they might well oppose changes. Likewise, some newer providers, such as PACE providers and palliative-care services, who are in tenuous positions because they are new, might well argue for perpetuation of their agenda even when a better option has already become available. The saving grace for change in this field might again be the oncoming remarkable increase in the population. For example, even if those facing fatal chronic illness used emergency rooms half as much, doubling the population would keep their rate of use constant.

This agenda is both urgent and incomplete. Urgency arises from the mandate created by avoidable current suffering and the prospect of worsening performance of the care system as the population ages. Trustworthy practices that are affordable, while achieving comfortable and meaningful living in the last years of life, would be a worthy promise to current citizens and a worthy legacy for the future.

Our agenda is yet incomplete. The data are thin, the mental models are new and incompletely tested, and the priorities and action steps will require ongoing learning to reshape them. Much is not yet known or understood. Perhaps the most important element in reform is to develop ways to garner insight and forge consensus that can fuel the will to make changes happen. Since interpreting facts and generating consensus require updating with new insights and emerging opportunities, the social structures that can do this work need to be enduring and ongoing. We also need many advocates and activists, and we need to have them push a shared agenda (Casarett, Karlawish, and Byock 2002).

Change is already seriously overdue. We have only two decades before the numbers with fatal chronic conditions will double. If we continue to do no better than we do now, the suffering will be overwhelming and the costs will be crippling. If we learn to do better and to deploy our knowledge effectively, we could instead live out our last years comfortably and meaningfully, with a care system that is sustainable, cost-effective, and politically popular.

Significant and enduring improvement in care for people with serious chronic illness requires leadership, analysis, and much hard work. Individuals and organizations must initiate efforts to learn how to serve those coming to the end of life and to translate those lessons into policy. All of us have a stake in this—all of us will reap the benefits if we learn to do it right; and all of us will endure unwarranted misery if we leave current shortcomings in place.

An Agenda for Action

Leaders and organizations that aim to help foment reforms can undertake important actions immediately. Here are some suggestions for the next few years, drawn from a variety of expert panels as well as from my experience (Eichner and Blumenthal 2003; Institute of Medicine 1997; Institute of Medicine 2001; Last Acts 2002; Smits, Furletti, and Vladeck 2002). If we get started, and learn from our early efforts, we will need to revise and restate this sort of list often.

Americans for Better Care of the Dying is a nonprofit educational organization dedicated to ensuring that all Americans can count on living comfortably and meaningfully despite serious chronic illnesses in the last years of life. The ABCD Web site at www.abcd-caring.org offers an online conversation about policy and various resources to support policy change. Updated insights and directions for reforms will be posted there.

Two members of the U.S. Congress, Jim Oberstar (D-Minn.) and Jim Ramstad (R-Minn.), have introduced a bill that could jump-start the process of reform. Although this bill does not propose the major reforms needed, it would build the infrastructure of understanding that could launch major changes. The main provisions of the bill are summarized in table 4.

Federal and State Policy Makers

Congress and at least some of the states would advance these issues dramatically if they directed public health agencies to gather data about the changing epidemiology of eventually fatal chronic illness. While much anecdotal evidence shows that the end of life is far from ideal for many patients, budget and programmatic decisions will be most effective when

Table 4. *Summary of Research and Demonstration Provisions in the Proposed "Living Well with Fatal Chronic Illness Act of 2003" (HR 2883)*

Department of Health and Human Services programs

- Research on how to adjust payment and regulations to ensure reliably good care
- Annual reports to Congress on new insights and changes to the quality of life for people with fatal chronic illness and their caregivers
- Medicare pilot programs to test innovations in service delivery

Health Resources and Services Administration

- Demonstrations of ways to improve the delivery of health care and support services
- Designation of persons with fatal chronic illnesses as a medically underserved population
- Training of health professionals, including palliative care and hospice

Agency for Healthcare Research and Quality

- Research concerning the merits and efficiencies of strategies for service delivery
- Coordination of innovation, evaluation, and service delivery relating to fatal chronic illness

Centers for Disease Control and Prevention

- Ongoing epidemiology of public experience of fatal chronic illness
- Inclusion of fatal chronic illness in public health, including response to emergency

National Institutes of Health

- Research, in each institute with fatal chronic illness in its purview, that focuses on understanding disability and suffering among patients with such illnesses
- Centers of excellence to conduct research, demonstrations, and education programs on fatal chronic illness and palliative care

Department of Veterans Affairs programs

- Studies through Geriatric Research, Education and Clinical Centers (GRECCs) and Health Services Research

- Additional professional training and staff development
- Cooperation with community service providers for home and hospice care
- Annual report on the status of veterans with fatal chronic illnesses and the department's research, education, and innovation activities

---

Source: Adapted from a summary of HR 2883 by Americans for Better Care of the Dying, www.abcd-caring.org.

based upon population-level data. Studies evaluating the experience of patients in different parts of the United States and from different socioeconomic backgrounds will provide a better understanding of those parts of the system most in need of reform and will also illustrate the relative merits of different ways of providing care. Epidemiologic data would also characterize how patients and their families live with worsening chronic illness, including both the financial and emotional impacts. Comparing findings across time and among similar populations would help target changes and measure quality.

Policy makers can also accelerate change by creating opportunities for innovation and then implementing strategies that show merit. Rather than the handful of Medicare-sponsored demonstrations now under way, there should be dozens of major trials. When an approach is shown to be effective and efficient, Medicare and Medicaid, at least, should design arrangements that ensure efficient and broad implementation. Policy makers and health-care administrators will have to be willing to rely upon the experiential learning of ongoing innovation and quality improvement, as well as evidence arising from rigorous research.

The coming crisis of caregiving may well make circumstances auspicious for the formation of politically popular agendas in innovations and reforms to support both paid workers and volunteer family caregivers. Political leaders would do well to engage in forming the political agenda for caregiving. Federal programs could pay at least the poorer family caregivers, provide training and respite for family caregivers, coordinate services and ensure career ladders for paid caregivers, and mandate health and disability insurance for most paid and full-time family caregivers.

Since most care in the last years of life is in public programs, and since quality and performance standards are already deficient and are likely to worsen with increasing costs and demands, an electorate aware of and angry over the shortcomings is exceedingly likely to appear at some point in the next few decades. This informed electorate will provide a political impetus for leaders who are ready with proposals, vision, and implementation. One troublesome arena will be revising expectations to accept the necessity of limits on some spending. Policy makers would do well to nourish and defend some efforts in this area, a challenge that is perhaps made more palatable by the considerations of competing comorbidities and limited life span that necessarily shape good decision making for those coming to the end of life.

Much of the care for fatal chronic illness depends upon Medicaid, which is partly funded and largely administered at the state level. State regulations and arrangements can make good care more possible or more difficult, and ongoing revisions to encourage good care are in order, just as with Medicare. In addition, state Medicaid directors have the opportunity for more substantial innovation in the dually eligible Medicaid/Medicare patients. PACE, for example, has given demonstrably good care and controlled costs, and its coherent funding makes creative strategies for services easy to implement. State waivers from conventional federal requirements can enable substantial innovation and learning. State programs could also take the lead in developing creative approaches to increasing the supply, support, and skills of caregivers.

Of course, this phase of life needs to be seen as a category that can and should be a target for tailored services. State and federal laws and regulations control many of the possibilities for good care. Various problematic elements have come to litter the terrain, arising around a particular troublesome case or in response to some systematic error. One recent review, for example, identified twenty states that have laws that make it more difficult to forego artificial nutrition and hydration than to make other medical treatment decisions (Sieger, Arnold, and Ahronheim 2002), even though the evidence is now good that artificial nutrition and hydration do not, on average, extend life, and all court cases have treated this decision like any other. This is the sort of artifact of old understanding that reforms should expunge.

PRIORITIES

· Establish epidemiology.
· Set up innovative service delivery.
· Define the category of serious, eventually fatal chronic illness.
· Encourage innovations in methods that equitably limit resource use.
· Support caregivers.

Public and Private Health-Care Purchasers or Insurers

Both the Medicare program and private purchasers of health care could demand results from providers, including the availability of coordinated, comprehensive care for patients living with serious, eventually fatal chronic illness. I have proposed that Medicare cut the payment to the hospital in half if the patient's stay is a repeat hospitalization for a serious, eventually fatal chronic illness and no advance care planning occurred on the first admission. That is the sort of proposal that would draw attention to the right issues, even if we only debated it and never implemented it.

What is of value to patients and families probably needs careful articulation, and then the priorities should conform to financial incentives. Purchasers also could improve professional caregivers' payment levels and job satisfaction and the support routinely provided to family caregivers. The Medicare program's existing efforts to improve beneficiary information could expand to address serious chronic illness and the end of life, including advance care planning and family caregiver support.

Private purchasers could also ensure that patients have adequate information about quality of care and about their choices for care when living with serious, eventually fatal chronic illness.

All funders, including employers, need to place a higher value on informal caregiving, including granting appropriate leave benefits to employees who must take time off to care for a dying family member.

PRIORITIES

· Link purchasing to quality.

· Define quality in terms of what is important to patients and family.

· Support both paid caregivers and family volunteer caregivers.

Federal Research Agencies

Federal government entities control most of the research funding that might reshape care delivery for the last phase of life. The Agency for Health Care Research and Quality, the Centers for Medicare and Medicaid Services, the Health Resources and Services Administration, the National Institutes of Health, the Department of Defense, and the Department of Veterans Affairs would do well to pursue research and demonstrations aimed at learning how to engineer an effective, efficient care system that can deliver reliable care (for example, to make the seven promises for every patient who lives with serious, eventually fatal illness, as described in chapter 5). The Medicare Payment Advisory Commission and the Medicare Coverage Advisory Committee might propose and test methods to restrain use of high-cost treatments that yield only small gains. Building on its success in managing the Ryan White Comprehensive AIDS Resources Emergency Act, the Health Resources and Services Administration (HRSA) could lead substantial work on care for eventually fatal conditions. Innovations in HRSA's hands could quickly teach how to implement better care strategies and to build the labor power and skills that an aging population will need, both in HRSA-sponsored clinics and in the care system generally. Increased development and dissemination of public information from federal health agencies, including HRSA and the Centers for Disease Control and Prevention, could begin to raise public awareness of issues surrounding fatal chronic conditions.

PRIORITIES

- Sponsor research and health services innovation.
- Develop and implement an epidemiology.
- Test methods for equitable allocation of limited resources.

Provider Organizations

Provider organizations need to improve the reliability and scope of their services, including relieving pain, making plans to avoid emergency responses to complications, and supporting family caregivers (Lynn 2000). The most effective techniques will include quality improvement (www.medicaring.org; Lynn, Schuster, and Kabcenell 2000; Lynn and Goldstein 2003) and increased accountability. Of course, raising the awareness of specialty groups and practitioners who do not yet recognize the problem will be an essential first step. Making public each provider system's own performance and making its promises explicit would also be worthy endeavors. Demonstrable excellence in small programs and areas provides goals and leadership in reform, so some providers should take on that role.

PRIORITIES

- Broadly implement rapid-cycle quality improvement.
- Innovate and measure results.
- Lead reform efforts.

Hospice and Palliative-Care Providers

Hospice and palliative-care program providers need to join in on reform and to judge the merits of particular changes in terms of the effects on those people who are approaching the end of life. The optimal roles for hospice and palliative care are undergoing definition and evolution. Those providers who have learned to provide good services and stay in business will be strongly tempted to adopt a holding pattern and resist further change. That would be unfortunate, in that it would unjustifiably slow the pace of adaptation to better serve the whole population. It is not clear whether the hospice of the future should focus upon the cancer trajectory patients or whether hospice programs can efficiently and effectively adapt to serve the other two trajectories. Likewise, evaluation of various strategies for providing and paying for palliative-care services (separate from hospice) will be essential to be sure that these services yield benefits worth their costs. The process of reform would yield better outcomes more quickly if innovation and evaluation yielded data, and if program and national leadership used those insights to guide reform.

PRIORITIES

- Advocate for population-based measures to guide change.
- Remain open to innovation, and avoid being limited to sustaining current practices.
- Press for evidence to guide reforms.

Individual Clinicians

Individual clinicians serving those with eventually fatal illness have an ongoing responsibility to improve personal practices, such as learning how best to communicate with and support seriously ill patients and families over time (Education for Physicians on End-of-Life Care Project 2000; Buckman 1993; Lo, Quill, and Tulsky 1999), how to make symptoms manageable (Doyle, Hanks, and MacDonald 1998), and how to help patients live fully within the constraints imposed by disease (Lynn and Harrold 1999). Providers also require additional training so that excellent care for this population is readily and reliably available. Not only do their clinical skills need ongoing improvement, but also they often need improved attitudes toward disability and death and increased familiarity with the ways that they can support the patient and family well. Just as for provider organizations, reform depends upon the presence of leaders who show that better performance is possible, so some physicians, nurses, social workers, chaplains, and others need to establish and report good practices. Probably the power and authority relationships of traditional medical practice will need alteration in order to create efficient and effective service-delivery models, since the leadership programs already established give nurses, social workers, and others a more central role than they have in the usual doctor's office or hospital. Individual professionals will need to adapt to change in order for reform to proceed.

PRIORITIES

· Enhance professionals' clinical skills.
· Train and encourage leadership.
· Learn and spread skills necessary for teamwork.

Family Caregivers

Family caregivers are often angry, isolated, and ignored, but many do find the work meaningful and probably most find it unavoidable. They will need to attend to patients' short-term needs and their own, but they also need to start to see that their situation is more demanding, more impoverishing, and more isolating than it needs to be—and that those shortcomings arise from policy decisions about the organization of and payment for care. Thus, whether during their time as caregivers or before or after, family caregivers need to find a strong voice for a better deal.

PRIORITIES

· Forge a strong political agenda for improved support, including payment, training, and respite.
· Set up communication vehicles among caregivers.
· Create a coherent political agenda.

Patients Living with Fatal Chronic Illness

A promising new level of consumerism is evident in the health-care arena (Institute for the Future 2000). Patients facing fatal chronic illness cannot take on the cause of reform; they have other priorities for their limited energies and limited time. However, they might often be able to make private choices in accord with evidence about quality. For example, *Handbook for Mortals* (Lynn and Harrold 1999, 88) advises patients facing the possibility of dying with shortness of breath to be sure that their doctor is competent and experienced in providing sedation at the end of life, or to change doctors. Patients could object to inadequate health care for the last part of life with the same level of outrage that they treat other obvious medical errors. The disorganized care arrangements that currently serve those coming to the end of life are rife with errors, and the patients might often have the awareness and energy to at least point out the shortcomings and tell their own stories.

PRIORITIES

· Choose providers on the basis of quality, including skills, reliability, and continuity.
· Report shortcomings.

Women's Groups

Women bear the brunt of serious chronic illness, first as caregivers and later as disabled persons. They are all too often isolated, impoverished, and in need. There is very little new-onset poverty in old age among men since, in general, they get free care from spouses and the couple has some savings. However, the second person to get sick enough to die is usually the woman, and she is often much more alone, much more impoverished, and older. Much more often, she has to pay for help, she comes to live in a nursing home, and she ends up dependent upon Medicaid for financing. The patterns are the outcome of social arrangements that link retirement income to peak earnings, do not value family caregiving, and make no allowance for the longer lives and longer span of disability in women.

PRIORITIES

- Galvanize around caregiving as the focus of reforms to benefit women.
- Insist upon Labor Department data about paid and unpaid caregiving, with regard to labor supply, compensation, retirement income, and working conditions.
- Pay family caregivers and ensure health and disability insurance.
- Pay fair wages for paid caregivers and give them reasonable working conditions and benefits.

Disease-Based, Faith-Based, Consumer Advocacy, and Professional Organizations

Advocacy groups that represent the issues most important to individuals coming toward the end of life are essential leaders in the overall agenda for change—educating policy makers about the needs of patients and the type of care to which they are entitled, demanding a better monitoring of the epidemiology of the last phase of life, and funding the needed studies. The poor, disabled, and sick are not politically powerful, and these three categories describe most of those facing fatal chronic illness. Advocacy groups will need to fill this vacuum, while ensuring that they solicit the input of those whose interests they represent. Several different types of advocacy organizations have a role to play, as each can bring to bear a unique focus and unique perspectives. These groups include those with a single disease or symptom focus (for instance, the American Cancer Society or the Pain Foundation), those representing particular types of health-care providers (such as the National Association for Home Care or the American Hospital Association), general senior citizen advocacy organizations (for example, the American Association of Retired Persons and the National Senior Citizens Law Center), and others. Since these groups must collaborate, they will have to develop ways to meet, network, and forge shared agendas for change.

Faith-based organizations may well take on the special role of addressing the difficult questions of meaningfulness in living in greatly limited circumstances toward the end of life. Religious traditions could be brought to bear on how to make meaningful interpretations of the experiences of patients and families facing dementia, profound and progressive disability, or unrelieved suffering.

The Last Acts Partnership (www.lastacts.org) helped to engender dozens of state-based partnerships to improve end-of-life care. Many of these groups focused mainly on public and professional education, but most have started working toward issues of public policy. Of the twenty-two state coalitions reported in 2002, half had worked on expanding Medicaid, on developing balanced policy on regulation of medications for pain, and on passing state laws on advance care planning (Last Acts 2003, at www.partnershipforcaring.org/statepolicy). This network is likely to change after its main sponsor, the Robert Wood Johnson Foundation, discontinues most of its support, though the current Rallying Points project continues to provide some services (www.rallyingpoints.org). However, the presence of a number of state-based coalitions could certainly be a strong point in addressing policy issues over time.

- · Establish broad mobilization.
- · Support a shared agenda.
- · Develop a cultural interpretation of meaningfulness of life near death.
- · Advocate for innovations and policy improvements in state Medicaid programs.

Philanthropic Organizations

Much innovation in this country depends first upon private foundations that can take on a risky proposal in a small program when federal research or clinical endeavors cannot. Philanthropic foundations have been very important in creating and moving an agenda for aging, disability, and dying. Those agendas have usually had the odd omission of not targeting the population of those who are very sick and disabled and who will die of their conditions, but whose main challenge is to live well for an uncertain but usually prolonged period. If there is to be a strong agenda for reform centered on this population, it will require the endorsement of philanthropics and probably their help in generating the agenda itself.

Until recently, two philanthropies had a strong hand in shaping the reforms in care for the last part of life. The Open Society Institute (a part of the Soros Foundation) established the Project on Death in America in 1995, which has assisted the development of a few hundred physicians, nurses, and social workers as leaders in the field and has sponsored a wide array of projects and innovations, from practical services to creative artists (www.soros.org/initiatives/pdia). The Robert Wood Johnson Foundation sponsored a series of projects, starting at about the same time, including small-scale innovations, state-based activist groups, and a communications campaign (www.rwjf.org/programs/infoByArea .jsp?value=End-of-Life+Care&id=000006). The Project on Death in America is closing in 2004, and the initiatives of the Robert Wood Johnson Foundation have also run their course, as the Last Acts communication vehicles have been merged with the existing issue organization Partnership for Caring, forming Last Acts Partnership (www .lastactspartnership.org/index_main.html).

The works sponsored by these two philanthropies, and a number of smaller contributors, have moved the field along, and their departure from active work in this arena will certainly mean that some important opportunities will be trimmed back. One might hope that other philanthropies or organizations focused upon a single disease (such as cancer, heart disease, Alzheimer's disease, or stroke) or organizations focused upon particular specialties or care settings (such as nursing homes, hospices, oncology, or geriatrics) would pick up the slack, but that has not happened. Some small initiatives in management of chronic disease have been launched, but even those have not tended to focus upon people with advanced stages or multiple conditions. Thus, 2004 marks a time of retrenchment rather than growth.

PRIORITIES

· Develop a creative, energetic, long-term agenda.
· Sponsor innovation and evaluation.
· Fund health services research.
· Encourage activist organizations.

News Media

Those who write, produce, and present the news must become more aware of the new epidemiology of dying and the implications for language, framing, and newsworthiness. Americans' view of what happens in the last years of life and how people can support one another and talk about meaningful events reflects the standard portrayals in the media. The situations they witness on television may mislead them about the typical outcomes of heroic procedures, such as cardiopulmonary resuscitation in dying patients (Diem, Lantos, and Tulsky 1996). While stories of medical miracles and prevention are popular, reports of the strength and tenacity of families enduring long disability before death are rare. Headlines could be changed from touting "lives saved" to reporting "deaths delayed," at least when the dying comes within a year or two despite the new development. Systems that allocate costly treatments in thoughtful ways could be the subject of respectful, intriguing reports, rather than condemnation for alleged rationing. Cultural change is difficult, but its urgent compression within the lifetime of the baby-boom generation is essential, to deal with a population that is mostly growing old and dying slowly. The news media cannot be far out in front of the willingness of the readers to adapt, but reporting need not lag behind the public's willingness to adopt new meanings either.

PRIORITIES

· Tell many stories of serious illness, family life, and dying.
· Frame them in honest ways.
· Adapt quickly to changing language and values.

Popular Culture

This culture has lived only half a century with most of us growing old before getting seriously ill, and living a long time with serious illness before dying. We have almost no tradition of interpretation, storytelling, or metaphor. Our movies about dying do not make heroes of the families of dementia patients; indeed, they do not even tell the stories of dementia patients. Our television shows do not show failed resuscitation or people who are living with serious illnesses who still have humor, perspective, and character. Popular culture has yet to address these new realities. Families confronted with years of dementia, disability from stroke, or frailty associated with advanced old age often simply have no idea what to expect, though they learn all too quickly how difficult the burdens are to bear and how even basic essential services are often uncoordinated, unreliable, and costly. A popular culture can hardly be "made to order," but it can be shaped. Among other elements, the portrayals of health care by writers, advertisers, producers, financiers, and actors could be more friendly to change and to adaptation, rather than more resistant.

PRIORITIES

- Try out many stories that describe experience and create metaphors and heroes.
- Discover what resonates with the public.
- Find the language that grants meaning to living with serious illness, in the eyes of the person whose life is about to close and in the eyes of those who are bound by ties of love and family.

References

42 CFR Part 418. Text from Code of Federal Regulations. Available from *Congressional Universe* online service. Bethesda, MD: Congressional Information Service. Available online at www.access.gpo.gov/nara/cfr/waisidx_00/42cfr418_00.html. Accessed February 2001.

Abel EK. 1990. Family care of the frail elderly. In Abel EK, Nelson MK, eds., *Circles of care: work and identity in women's lives*, 65–91. Albany, NY: State University of New York Press.

Administration on Aging. 2003. Family caregiving. Available online at www.aoa.gov. Accessed November 2003.

Agency for Healthcare Research and Quality. 2003. *National healthcare quality report.* Rockville, MD: U.S. Department of Health and Human Services. Available online at www.qualitytools.ahrq.gov/qualityreport. Accessed February 2004.

Alemayehu B, Warner KE. 2004. The lifetime distribution of health care costs. *Health Serv Res.* 39:627–642.

Alzheimer's Association. 2001. Frequently asked questions about Alzheimer's disease. Available online at www.alz.org/ResourceCenter/FactSheets/FSAlzheimerStats.pdf. Accessed July 2003.

American Geriatrics Society. 1997. Measuring quality of care at the end of life: a statement of principles. *J Am Geriatr Soc.* 45:526–527. Available online at www.americangeriatrics.org/products/positionpapers/quality.shtml. Accessed February 2004.

American Hospital Association. 2001. TrendWatch. Available online at www.aha.org.

———. 2002. Circle of Life awards. Available online at www.hospitalconnect.com/aha/awards-events/circle_of_life/index.html. Accessed July 2003.

American Pain Society. 1995. Quality improvement guidelines for the treatment of acute pain and cancer. *JAMA.* 274:1874–1880.

Americans for Better Care of the Dying. 1999. Study shows Oregon's Physician Orders for Life-Sustaining Treatment (POLST) document prevents unwanted interventions. *ABCD Exchange.* January. Available online at www.abcd-caring.org/newsletter.htm. Accessed November 2003.

———. 2001. Improving care for veterans with heart and lung disease: award-winning East Orange VAMC team solves problems in care systems. *ABCD Exchange*. May-June. Available online at www.abcd-caring.org/newsletter .htm. Accessed December 2002.

Anderson G, Horvath J, Anderson C. 2002. Chronic conditions: making the case for ongoing care. Baltimore, MD: Partnership for Solutions, Johns Hopkins University. Available online at www.partnershipforsolutions.org/DMS/ files/chronicbook2002.pdf. Accessed February 2004.

Arno PS, Levine C, Memmott MM. 1999. The economic value of informal caregiving. *Health Affairs*. 18:182–188.

Assistant Secretary for Planning and Evaluation and Administration on Aging. 1998. Informal caregiving: compassion in action. Washington, DC: Government Printing Office. Available online at http://aspe.hhs.gov/search/ daltcp/reports/Carebr02.pdf. Accessed February 2004.

Atchley RC. 1996. Frontline workers in long-term care: recruitment, retention, and turnover issues in an era of rapid growth. Oxford, OH: Scripps Gerontology Center at Miami University.

Baer WM, Hanson LC. 2000. Families' perception of the added value of hospice in the nursing home. *J Am Geriatr Soc*. 48:879–882.

Barnato AE, Kagay CR, McClellan MB, Garber AM. 2004. Trends in inpatient treatment intensity among Medicare beneficiaries at the end of life. *Health Serv Res*. 39(2):359–372.

Bartlett DF. 1999. The new healthcare consumer. *J Health Care Fin*. 25:44–51.

Berenson RA, Horvath J. 2003. Confronting the barriers to chronic care management in Medicare. *Health Affairs*. W3-37–W3-53. Web exclusive. Available online at http://content.healthaffairs.org/cgi/content/full/hlthaff.w3 .37v1/DC1. Accessed February 2004.

Bernabei R, Gambassi G, Lapane K, Landi F, Gatsonis C, Dunlop R, Lipsitz L, Steel K, Mor V. 1998. Management of pain in elderly with cancer: SAGE study group systematic assessment of geriatric drug use via epidemiology. *JAMA*. 279:1877–1882.

Berwick, DM. 1996. Quality comes home. *Ann Intern Med*. 125:839–843.

———. 1999. Twenty improvements in end of life care: changes internists could do next week! Keynote address at the American College of Physicians–American Society of Internal Medicine (ACP-ASIM) annual meeting, April 22. Available online at www.abcd-caring.org/tools/intern.htm. Accessed July 2003.

Biegel DE, Sales E, Schulz R. 1991. *Family caregiving in chronic illness*. Thousand Oaks, CA: Sage Publications.

Billings JA, Block S. 1997. Palliative care in undergraduate medical education: status report and future directions. *JAMA*. 278:733–738.

Bird CE, Shugarman LR, Lynn J. 2002. Age and gender differences in health care utilization and spending for Medicare beneficiaries in their last years of life. *J Palliat Med*. 5:705–712.

Bodenheimer T, Lorig K, Holman H, Grumbach K. 2002. Patient self-management of chronic disease in primary care. *JAMA*. 288:2469-2475.

Bodenheimer T, Wagner EH, Grumbach K. 2002a. Improving primary care for patients with chronic illness. *JAMA*. 288:1775–1779.

———. 2002b. Improving primary care for patients with chronic illness: the chronic care model, part 2. *JAMA*. 288:1909–1914.

Bookbinder M. 2001. Raising the standard of care for imminently dying patients using quality improvement: an interview with Marilyn Bookbinder. *Innovations in End-of-Life Care*. 3(4). Available online at www2.edc.org/lastacts/archives/archivesJuly01/bbfeatureinn.asp. Accessed February 2004.

Boult C, Kane RL, Brown R. 2000. Managed care of chronically ill older people: the U.S. experience. *BMJ*. 321:1011–1014.

Boult C, Rassen J, Rassen A, Moore R, Robinson S. 2000. The effects of case management on the costs of health care for enrollees in Medicare+Choice plans: a randomized trial. *J Am Geriatr Soc*. 48:996–1001.

Breaux J. 2002. Broken and unsustainable: the cost of long-term care for baby boomers. Opening statement, U.S. Senate Special Committee on Aging hearing, March 21. Available online at http://aging.senate.gov/events/032102.html. Accessed July 2003.

Brock DB, Foley DJ. 1998. Demography and epidemiology of dying in the U.S., with emphasis on deaths of older persons. *Hospice J*. 13:49–60.

Brumley RD, Enguidanos S, Cherin DA. 2003. Effectiveness of a home-based palliative care program for end-of-life. *J Palliat Med*. 6:715–724.

Buckman R. 1993. *How to break bad news: a guide for health care professionals*. Toronto: University of Toronto Press.

Butler R, Meier D, Nyberg J. 2003. Palliative care academic career awards: a public-private partnership to improve care for the most vulnerable. New York: International Longevity Center. Available online at www.ilcusa.org/_lib/pdf/palliativecare.pdf. Accessed February 2004.

Byock I. 2000. Completing the continuum of cancer care: integrating life-prolongation and palliation. *Ca Cancer J Clin*. 50(2):123–132.

Callahan D. 1995. Frustrated mastery: the cultural context of death in America. *West J Med*. 163:226–230.

————. 1998. *False hopes: overcoming the obstacles to a sustainable, affordable medicine*. New Brunswick, NJ: Rutgers University Press.

Callahan J. 2001. Police perspectives on workforce issues and care of older people. *Generations*. 25(1):12–16.

Campbell DE, Lynn J, Louis TA, Shugarman L. 2004. Medicare program costs associated with hospice use. *Ann Intern Med*. 140:269–277.

Campbell ML, Frank RR. 1997. Experience with an end-of-life practice at a university hospital. *Crit Care Med*. 25:197–202.

Carron AT, Lynn J, Keaney P. 1999. End-of-life care in medical textbooks. *Ann Intern Med*. 130:82–86.

Casarett DJ, Karlawish JHT, Byock I. 2002. Advocacy and activism: missing pieces in the quest to improve end-of-life care. *J Palliat Med*. 5:3–12.

Casarett D, Karlawish JHT, Sugarman J. 2000. Determining when quality improvement initiatives should be considered research: proposed criteria and potential implications. *JAMA*. 283:2275–2280.

Cassel CK, Foley KM. 1999. *Principles for care of patients at the end of life: an emerging consensus among the specialties of medicine*. New York, NY: Milbank Memorial Fund.

Catholic Health Association. 2003. PACE success to date. Available online at www.chausa.org/longterm/ltpace.asp. Accessed July 2003.

Center for Medicare and Medicaid Services. 2002. Combined trustees report. Available online at http://cms.hhs.gov/publications/trusteesreport/2002. Accessed July 2003.

Centers for Disease Control and Prevention (CDC). 1999. Achievements in public health, 1900–1999: changes in the public health system. *Morbidity and Mortality Weekly Report* 48:1141–1147.

————. 2002a. About CDC: CDC's mission. Available online at www.cdc.gov/aboutcdc.htm. Accessed February 2004.

————. 2002b. *The burden of chronic diseases and their risk factors*. Available online at www.cdc.gov/nccdphp/burdenbook2002/index.htm. Accessed July 2003.

Center to Advance Palliative Care (CAPC). 2000a. The case for hospital-based palliative care. Available online at www.capc.org/Files/tmp_133221135.pdf. Accessed July 2003.

————. 2000b. Planning a hospital-based palliative care program: a primer for institutional leaders. Technical assistance series. Available online at www.capc.org/Files/tmp_133221516.pdf. Accessed July 2003.

————. 2003. FAQs online. Available online at www.capc.org/site_root/FAQs#faq_119115305.html. Accessed November 2003.

Chen A, Brown R, Archibald N, Aliotta S, Fox P. 2000. Best practices in coordinated care. Final report to the Health Care Financing Administration. Contract no. 500–95–0084(04). Princeton, NJ: Mathematica Policy Research, Inc.

Christakis NA. 1999. *Death foretold: prophecy and prognosis in medical care.* Chicago: University of Chicago Press.

Citizens for Long-Term Care. 2003. *Long-term care financing and the long-term care workforce crisis: causes and solutions.* Washington, DC: Paraprofessional Healthcare Institute.

Claessens MT, Lynn J, Zhong Z, Desbiens NA, Phillips RS, Wu AW, Harrell FE Jr, Connors AF Jr . 2000. Dying with lung cancer or chronic obstructive pulmonary disease: insights from SUPPORT. *J Am Geriatr Soc.* 48: S146–153.

Cleeland CS, Gonin R, Hatfield AD, Edmonson JH, Blum RH, Stewart JA, Pandya KJ. 1994. Pain and its treatment in outpatients with metastatic cancer. *N Engl J Med.* 330:592–596.

Cleeland CS, Reyes-Gibby CC, Schall M, Nolan K, Paice J, Rosenberg JM, Tollett JH, Kerns RD. 2003. Rapid improvement in pain management: the Veterans Health Administration and the Institute for Healthcare Improvement Collaborative. *Clin J Pain.* 19:298–305.

Coleman EA, Grothaus LC, Sandhu N, Wagner EH. 1999. Chronic care clinics: a randomized controlled trial of a new model of primary care for frail older adults. *J Am Geriatr Soc.* 47:775–783.

Collins KS, Hughes DL, Doty MM, Ives BL, Edwards JN, Tenney K. 2002. Diverse communities, common concerns: addressing health care quality for minority Americans. New York: The Commonwealth Fund. Available online at www.cmwf.org/programs/minority/collins_diversecommunities_523.pdf. Accessed November 2003.

Congressional Budget Office. 1999. CBO memorandum: projections of expenditures for long-term care services for the elderly. Washington, DC. Available online at www.cbo.gov/showdoc.cfm?index=1123. Accessed July 2003.

Cook A. 1999. Strategies for containing drug costs: implications for a Medicare benefit. *Health Care Financ Rev.* 20(3):9. Available online at http://cms.hhs.gov/review/99Spring/cook.pdf. Accessed July 2003.

Cornoni-Huntley JC, Foley DJ, White LR, Suzman R, Berkman LF, Evans DA, Wallace RB. 1985. Epidemiology of disability in the oldest old: methodologic issues and preliminary findings. *Milbank Mem Fund Q Health Soc.* 63(2): 350–376.

Corti MC, Guralnik JM, Salive ME, Sorkin JD. 1994. Serum albumin and physical disability as predictors of mortality in older persons. *JAMA*. 272: 1036–1042.

Covinsky KE, Goldman L, Cook EF, Oye R, Desbiens N, Reding D, Fulkerson W, Connors AF Jr, Lynn J, Phillips RS. 1994. The impact of serious illness on patients' families. *JAMA*. 272:1939–1944.

Coyle N. 1997. Interdisciplinary collaboration in hospital palliative care: chimera or goal? *Palliat Med*. 11:265–266.

Crimmins EM, Saito Y, Reynolds SL. 1997. Further evidence on recent trends in the prevalence and incidence of disability among older Americans from two sources: the LSOA and the NHIS. *J Gerontol B Psychol Sci Soc Sci*. 52:S59–71.

Crippen DL. 2002. Disease management in Medicare: data analysis and benefit design issues. Congressional Budget Office testimony before the Special Committee on Aging, U.S. Senate. September 19. Washington, DC: Congressional Budget Office. Available online at www.cbo.gov/showdoc .cfm?index=3776&sequence=0. Accessed February 2004.

Dartmouth Atlas of Health Care. 1998. *Dartmouth atlas of health care in the United States*. Wennberg JE, Cooper M, eds. Chicago: American Hospital Association Press. Available online at www.dartmouthatlas.org/atlaslinks/ 98atlas.php. Accessed November 2002.

———. 1999. *The quality of medical care in the United States: a report on the medical program*. Wennberg JE, ed. Chicago: American Hospital Association Press. Available online at www.dartmouthatlas.org/tables/99table7.php. Accessed February 2004

Davis RM, Wagner EH, Groves T. 2000. Advances in managing chronic disease. *BMJ*. 320:525–526.

Desai M, Pratt LA, Lentzner H, Robinson KN. 2001. Trends in vision and hearing among older Americans. Aging trends, no. 2. Hyattsville, MD: Centers for Disease Control and Prevention, National Center on Health Statistics. Available online at www.cdc.gov/nchs/data/agingtrends/02vision.pdf. Accessed February 2004.

Diem SJ, Lantos JD, Tulsky JA. 1996. Cardiopulmonary resuscitation on television: miracles and misinformation. *N Engl J Med*. 13:1578–1582.

Doyle D, Hanks GWC, MacDonald N, eds. 1998. *Oxford textbook of palliative medicine*. 2nd ed. New York: Oxford University Press.

Dubler NN, Bellin E. 2001. The quality improvement–research divide and the need for external oversight. *Am J Public Health*. 91:1512–1517.

Dunn PM, Schmidt TA, Carley MM, Donius M, Weinstein MA, Dull VT. 1996.

A method to communicate patient preferences about medically indicated life-sustaining treatment in the out-of-hospital setting. *J Am Geriatr Soc.* 44:785–791. Available online at www.ohsu.edu/ethics/polstabstracts.htm. Accessed July 2003.

Du Pen SL, Du Pen AR, Polissar N, Hansberry J, Kraybill BM, Stillman M, Panke J, Everly R, Syrjala K. 1999. Implementing guidelines for cancer pain management: results of a randomized controlled trial. *J Clin Oncol.* 17:361–370.

Education for Physicians on End-of-Life Care (EPEC) Project. 2000. Available online at www.EPEC.net. Accessed July 2003.

Eichner J, Blumenthal D, eds. 2003. *Medicare in the twenty-first century: building a better chronic care system.* Washington, DC: National Academy of Social Insurance.

Emanuel EJ, Ash A, Yu W, Gazelle G, Levinsky NG, Saynina O, McClellan M, Moskowitz M. 2002. Managed care, hospice use, site of death, and medical expenditures in the last year of life. *Arch Intern Med.* 162:1722–1728.

Emanuel EJ, Young-Xu Y, Levinsky NG, Gazelle G, Saynina O, Ash AS. 2003. Chemotherapy use among Medicare beneficiaries at the end of life. *Ann Intern Med.* 138:639–643.

Employee Benefit Research Institute. 1997. National health care expenditures, 1995. In *EBRI databook on employee benefits.* 4th ed. Available online at www.ebri.org/facts/0397fact.htm. Accessed July 2003.

———. 2002. Income of Kansas retirees won't keep pace with expenses, new research concludes. Available online at www.ebri.org/prrel/pr605.htm. Accessed July 2003.

End-of-Life Nursing Education Consortium (ELNEC). 2000. About ELNEC. Available online at www.aacn.nche.edu/elnec/. Accessed July 2003.

End of Life/Palliative Education Resource Center (EPERC). 2001. Available online at www.eperc.mcw.edu/about/start.cfm. Accessed July 2003.

Evans DA, Funkenstein HH, Albert MS, Scherr PA, Cook NR, Chown MJ, Hebert LE, Hennekens CH, Taylor JO. 1989. Prevalence of Alzheimer's disease in a community population of older persons: higher than previously reported. *JAMA.* 262:2552–2556.

Federal Interagency Forum on Aging. 2000. Older Americans: key indicators of well being. Related statistics. Available online at www.agingstats.gov/chartbook2000/population.html. Accessed July 2003.

Feldman PH. 1997. Labor market issues in home care. In Fox DM, Raphael C, eds., *Home-based care for a new century,* 155–184. Malden, MA: Blackwell Publishers.

Ferrell B. 1998. The family. In Doyle D, Hanks GWC, MacDonald N, eds., *The Oxford textbook of palliative medicine*, 909–918. 2nd ed. London: Oxford University Press.

Ferrell B, Virani R, Grant M, Juarez G. 2000. Analysis of palliative care content in nursing textbooks. *J Pall Care.* 16:39–47.

Fisher ES, Wennberg DE, Stukel TA, Gottlieb DJ, Lucas FL, Pinder EL. 2003a. The implications of regional variations in Medicare spending. Part 1: the content, quality, and accessibility of care. *Ann Intern Med.* 138:273–287.

———. 2003b. The implications of regional variations in Medicare spending. Part 2: health outcomes and satisfaction with care. *Ann Intern Med.* 138: 288–298.

Fox D. 1993. *Power and illness: the failure and future of American health policy.* Berkeley: University of California Press.

Fox E, Landrum-McNiff K, Zhong Z, Dawson NV, Wu AW, Lynn J. 1999. Evaluation of prognostic criteria for determining hospice eligibility in patients with advanced lung, heart, or liver disease. SUPPORT investigators. *JAMA.* 282:1638–1645.

Freedman VA, Aykan H, Martin LG. 2001. Aggregate changes in severe cognitive impairment among older Americans: 1993 and 1998. *J Gerontol B Psychol Sci Soc Sci.* 56:S100–111.

Freedman VA, Martin LG. 1998. Understanding trends in functional limitations among older Americans. *Am J Public Health.* 88:1457–1462.

Freedman VA, Martin LG, Schoeni RF. 2002. Recent trends in disability and functioning among older adults in the United States: a systematic review. *JAMA.* 288:3137–3146.

Fried LP, Guralnik M. 1997. Disability in older adults: evidence regarding significance, etiology, and risk. *J Am Geriatr Soc.* 45:92–100.

Fried LP, Tangen CM, Walston J, Newman AB, Hirsch C, Gottdiener J, Seeman T, Tracy R, Kop WJ, Burke G, McBurnie MA. 2001. Frailty in older adults: evidence for a phenotype. *J Gerontol.* 56A:M146–156.

Fried TR, van Doorn C, O'Leary JR, Tinetti ME, Drickamer MA. 1999. Older persons' preferences for site of terminal care. *Ann Intern Med.* 131:109–112.

Friss L. 1993. Family caregivers as case managers: a statewide model for enhancing consumer choice. *J Case Mgmt.* 2:53–58.

Gage B, Dao T. 2000. Medicare's hospice benefit: use and expenditures, 1996 cohort. Prepared for the U.S. Department of Health and Human Services. March. Available online at www.aspe.hhs.gov/daltcp/reports/96useexp.htm. Accessed February 2004.

Gallup Organization. 1996. Knowledge and attitudes related to hospice care. Prepared for the National Hospice Organization.

Gillick MR. 2001. Pinning down frailty. *J Gerontol.* 56A:M134–135.

———. 2004. Medicare coverage for technological innovations—time for new criteria? *N Engl J Med.* 350:2199–2203.

Gostin LO. 2003. At law: the judicial dismantling of the Americans with Disabilities Act. *Hastings Center Report.* March-April. 33(2):9–12.

Greene HL. 2000. The implantable cardioverter-defibrillator. *Clin Card.* 23:315–326.

Groth-Juncker A, McCusker J. 1983. Where do elderly patients prefer to die? *J Am Geriatr Soc.* 31:457–461.

Gruenberg L, Kaganova J. 1997. *An examination of the cost-effectiveness of PACE in relation to Medicare.* Cambridge, MA: DataChron Health Systems, Inc.

Hammes BJ. 2001. What does it take to help adults successfully plan for future medical decisions? *J Palliat Med.* 4:453–456.

Hammes BJ, Rooney BL. 1998. Death and end of life planning in one midwestern community. *Arch Intern Med.* 158:383–390.

Hanrahan P, Raymond M, McGowan E, Luchins DJ. 1999. Criteria for enrolling dementia patients in hospice: a replication. *Am J Hosp Pall Care.* 16:395–400.

Health Resources and Services Administration. 2003. Projected supply, demand, and shortages of registered nurses: 2000–2020. Available online at http://hrsa.gov/healthworkforce/rnproject/default.htm. Accessed November 2003.

Himes CL. 1992. Future caregivers: projected family structures of older persons. *J Geron Soc Sci* 47:S17–26.

Himmelstein DU, Lewontin JP, Woolhandler S. 1996. Medical employment in the United States, 1968–1993: the importance of health sector jobs for African Americans and women. *Am J Public Health.* 86:525–528.

Hoffman C, Rice DP. 1995. Estimates based on the 1987 National Medical Expenditure Survey. University of California, San Francisco, Institute for Health and Aging.

Hogan C. 2001. Medicare beneficiaries' access to hospice services in rural areas: an initial analysis. Report to the Medicare Payment Advisory Commission. June 14. Washington, DC.

Hogan C, Lynn J, Gabel J, Lunney J, Mara A, Wilkinson A. 2000. Medicare beneficiaries' costs and use of care in the last year of life. Report by the Medicare Payment Advisory Commission, MedPAC no. 00–1. Washington, DC.

Hoover DR, Crystal S, Kumar R, Sambamoorthi U, Cantor JC. 2002. Medical expenditures during the last year of life: findings from the 1992–1996 Medicare Current Beneficiary Survey. *Health Serv Res.* 37(6):1625–1642.

Hooyman NR, Kiyak HA. 1996. *Social Gerontology.* 4th ed. Boston: Allyn and Bacon.

Innovations in End-of-Life Care. 2000. AHA's Circle of Life award: an overview of nine programs honored. May-June. Education Development Center, Inc. Available online at www2.edc.org/lastacts/archives/archivesMay00/circle.asp. Accessed November 2003.

———. 2002. Executive summary of 2002 Circle of Life award winner. June. Education Development Center, Inc. Available online at www2.edc.org/lastacts/archives/archivesJuly02/safeconduct.asp. Accessed November 2003.

Institute for Health and Aging. 1996. University of California, San Francisco. *Chronic care in America: a twenty-first century challenge.* Princeton, NJ: Robert Wood Johnson Foundation.

Institute for the Future. 2000. *Health and healthcare 2010: the forecast, the challenge.* San Francisco: Jossey-Bass.

Institute of Medicine (IOM). 1997. *Approaching death: improving care at the end of life.* Committee on Care at the End of Life, Institute of Medicine. Field MJ, Cassel CK, eds. Washington, DC: National Academies Press.

———. 1999a. *Definition of serious and complex medical conditions.* Committee on Serious and Complex Medical Conditions, Institute of Medicine. Chrvala CA, Sharfstein S, eds. Washington, DC: National Academies Press.

———. 1999b. *To err is human: building a safer health care system.* Committee on Quality of Health Care in America, Institute of Medicine. Kohn L, Corrigan J, Donaldson MS, eds. Washington, DC: National Academies Press.

———. 2001. *Crossing the quality chasm: a new health system for the twenty-first century.* Committee on Quality of Health Care in America, Institute of Medicine, ed. Washington, DC: National Academies Press.

———. 2002. *Fostering rapid advances in health care: learning from system demonstrations.* Committee on Rapid Advance Demonstration Projects: Health Care Finance and Delivery Systems, Institute of Medicine. Corrigan J, Greiner A, Erickson S, eds. Washington, DC: National Academies Press.

———. 2003. *Priority areas for national action: transforming health care quality.* Committee on Identifying Priority Areas for Quality Improvement, Institute of Medicine. Adams K, Corrigan J, eds. Washington, DC: National Academies Press.

———. 2004. Quality chasm summit: invitational summit meeting. Washington, DC. January 6–7.

Jacoby MB, Sullivan TA, Warren E. 2001. Rethinking the debates over health care financing: evidence from the bankruptcy courts. *New York University Law Rev.* 76:375–418.

Joint Commission on Accreditation of Healthcare Organizations (JCAHO). 2001. Pain assessment and management standards for 2001. Available online at www.jcrinc.com/subscribers/printview.asp?durki=3243. Accessed July 2003.

Kane RL, Kane RA. 2001. Emerging issues in chronic care. In Binstock RH, George LK, eds., *Handbook of aging and the social sciences*, 406–419. 5th ed. San Diego: Academic Press.

Kassner E, Bectel R. 1998. Midlife and older Americans with disabilities: who gets help? Public Policy Institute. Washington, DC: American Association of Retired Persons. Available online at http://research.aarp.org/il/d16883_midlife_1.html. Accessed February 2004.

Kaye S, LaPlante MP, Carlson D, Wenger BL. 1996. Trends in disability rates in the United States, 1970–1994. National Institute on Disability and Rehabilitation research report. Washington, DC: U.S. Department of Health and Human Services. Available online at http://dsc.ucsf.edu/UCSF/pub. Accessed February 2004.

Kendall DB, Tremain K, Lemieux J, Levine SR. 2003. *Healthy aging v. chronic illness: preparing Medicare for the new health care challenge*. Washington, DC: Progressive Policy Institute.

Kennedy, M. 1998. Baby boomers likely to go out with a bang. *Wisc Med J.* 97(11):24–27.

Kiecolt-Glaser J, Glaser R, Gravenstein S, Malarkey W, Sheridan J. 1996. Chronic stress alters the immune response to influenza virus vaccine in older adults. *Proc Natl Acad Sci USA.* 93:3043–3047.

Kinsella K, Velkoff V. 2001. An aging world: 2001. U.S. Census Bureau series P95/01–1. Washington, DC: Government Printing Office.

Knaus WA, Harrell FE, Lynn J, Goldman L, Phillips RS, Connors AF Jr, Dawson NV, Fulkerson WJ Jr, Califf RM, Desbiens N, et al. 1995. The SUPPORT prognostic model: objective estimates of survival for seriously ill hospitalized adults. *Ann Intern Med.* 122:191–203.

Koffman J, Snow P. 2001. Informal carers of dependants with advanced disease. In Addington-Hall JM, Higginson I, eds., *Palliative care for non-cancer patients*. London: Oxford University Press.

Kübler-Ross E. 1969. *On death and dying*. New York: Simon and Schuster. Reprint, 1997.

Last Acts. 1997. Precepts of palliative care. Task Force on Palliative Care.

Princeton, NJ: Robert Wood Johnson Foundation. Available online at www.lastacts.org/docs/profprecepts.pdf. Accessed July 2003.

———. 2000. Champion for improving end-of-life care. News release. Available online at www.lastacts.org/statsite/3657La%5Fmrc%5Fnewsrelease.html. Accessed November 2003.

———. 2002. Means to a better end: a report on dying in America today. Available online at www.lastacts.org/files/misc/meansfull.pdf. Accessed November 2003.

———. 2003. State initiatives in end-of-life care. Issue 19. Kansas City: Midwest Bioethics Center. Available online at www.lastacts.org/files/publications/coalition_final.pdf. Accessed February 2004.

Levine C. 1999. The loneliness of the long-term care giver. *N Engl J Med.* 340:1587–1590.

———. 2003. Making room for family caregivers: seven innovative hospital programs. United Hospital Fund special report. New York: United Hospital Fund of New York. Available online at www.uhfnyc.org/pubs-stories3220/pubs-stories_show.htm?doc_id=156825. Accessed February 2004.

Levine C, Kuerbis AN, Gould DA, Navalie-Waliser M, Feldman PH, Donelan K. 2000. A survey of family caregivers in New York City: findings and implications for the health care system. New York: Visiting Nurse Service of New York and United Hospital Fund of New York. Available online at www.uhfnyc.org/pubs-stories3220/pubs-stories_show.htm?doc_id = 97890. Accessed February 2004.

Liao Y, McGee DL, Cao G, Cooper PR. 2000. Quality of the last year of life of older adults: 1986 vs 1993. *JAMA.* 283:512–518.

Lo B, Groman M. 2003. Oversight of quality improvement: focusing on benefits and risks. *Arch Intern Med.* 163:1481–1486.

Lo B, Quill T, Tulsky J. 1999. Discussing palliative care with patients. American College of Physicians–American Society of Internal Medicine (ACP-ASIM) End-of-Life Care Consensus Panel. *Ann Intern Med.* 130:744–749.

Lorig KR, Sobel DS, Stewart AL, Brown BW Jr, Bandura A, Ritter P, Gonzalez VM, Laurent DD, Holman HR. 1999. Evidence suggesting that a chronic disease self-management program can improve health status while reducing hospitalization: a randomized trial. *Med Care.* 37:5–14.

Loxtercamp D. 1996. Hearing voices: how should doctors respond to their calling? *N Engl J Med.* 335:1991–1993.

Lubitz J, Cai L, Kramarow E, Lentzner H. 2003. Health, life expectancy, and health care spending among the elderly. *N Engl J Med.* 349:1048–1055.

Lubitz J, Riley G. 1993. Trends in Medicare payments in the last year of life. *N Engl J Med.* 328:1092–1096.

Lunney JR. 2000. Resources for caregivers of terminally ill cancer patients. *Cancer Pract.* 8:99–100.

Lunney JR, Lynn J, Foley DJ, Lipson S, Guralnik JM. 2003. Patterns of functional decline at the end of life. *JAMA.* 289:2387–2392.

Lunney JR, Lynn J, Hogan C. 2002. Profiles of older Medicare decedents. *J Am Geriatr Soc.* 50:1108–1112.

Lynch Schuster J. 1999. Veterans Health Administration's addition of pain as a fifth vital sign may have far-reaching effects. *Washington Post.* February 1.

———. 2002. Senators recommend ways to secure financial future of family caregivers. *ABCD Exchange.* 11(22). Available online at www.abcd-caring .org/newsletter.htm. Accessed February 2004.

Lynn J. 2000. Quality of life at the end of life. *JAMA.* 284:1513–1515.

———. 2001. Serving patients who may die soon and their families. *JAMA.* 285:925–932.

———. 2004. When does quality improvement count as research? Human subject protection and theories of knowledge. *Quality Safety and Healthcare.* 13:67–70.

Lynn J, Adamson D. 2003. RAND Corporation. *Living well at the end of life: adapting health care to serious chronic illness in old age.* White paper. Washington, DC: RAND Corporation. Available online at www.rand.org/ publications/WP/WP137. Accessed February 2004.

Lynn J, Blanchard J, Campbell D, Jayes RL, Lunney J. 2002. The last three years of life through Medicare claims review. Society for General Internal Medicine abstract. 17(S1):203.

Lynn J, Cretin S. 2000. After aging [editorial]. *J Am Geriatr Soc.* 48: 1017–1018.

Lynn J, Goldstein N. 2003. Advance care planning for fatal chronic illness: tolerating mistakes as the standard of practice. *Ann Intern Med.* 138:812–818.

Lynn J, Harrell FE, Cohn F, Hamel MB, Dawson N, Wu AW. 1996. Defining the "terminally ill": insights from SUPPORT. *Duquesne L Rev.* 35:311–335.

Lynn J, Harrell F, Cohn F, Wagner D, Connors AF. 1997. Prognoses of seriously ill hospitalized patients on the days before death: implications for patient care and public policy. *New Horiz.* 5:56–61.

Lynn J, Harrold J. 1999. *Handbook for mortals.* New York: Oxford University Press.

Lynn J, Harrold JK, Ayers E. 1997. A good death: improving care inch-by-inch. *Bioethics Forum.* 13:38–40.

Lynn J, Nolan K, Kabcenell A, Weissman D, Milne C, Berwick DM. 2002. Reforming care for persons near the end of life: the promise of quality improvement. *Ann Intern Med.* 137:117–122.

Lynn J, O'Connor MA, Dulac JD, Roach MJ, Ross C, Wasson J. 1999. MediCaring: development and test marketing of a supportive care benefit for older people. *J Am Geriatr Soc.* 47:1058–1064.

Lynn J, Schall M, Milne C, Nolan K, Kabcenell A. 2000. Quality improvements in end of life care: insights from two collaboratives. *Joint Commn J Qual Impr.* 26:254–267.

Lynn J, Schuster JL, Kabcenell A. 2000. *Improving care for the end of life: a sourcebook for health care managers and clinicians.* New York: Oxford University Press.

Lynn J, Wilkinson A, Etheredge L. 2001. Financing of care for fatal chronic disease: opportunities for Medicare reform. *West J Med.* 175:299–302.

Macmillan Cancer Relief. 2004. Gold Standards Framework. Available online at www.macmillan.org.uk/healthprofessionals/disppage.asp?id=2062. Accessed February 2004.

Mann WC. 2001. The potential of technology to ease the care provider's burden. *Generations.* 25(1):44–48.

Manton KG, Corder LS, Stallard E. 1993. Estimates of change in chronic disability and institutional incidence and prevalence rates in the U.S. elderly population from the 1982, 1984, and 1989 National Long Term Care Survey. *J Gerontol Soc Sci.* 48:S153–166.

———. 1997. Chronic disability trends in elderly United States populations: 1982–1994. *Proc Natl Acad Sci.* 94:2593–2598.

Manton KG, Gu X. 2001. Changes in the prevalence of chronic disability in the United States black and nonblack population above age 65 from 1982–1999. *Proc Natl Acad Sci.* 98:6354–6359.

Marmor T. 2000. *The politics of Medicare.* 2nd ed. New York: Aldine De Gruyter.

Maxwell S, Moon M, Segal M. 2001. Growth in Medicare and out-of-pocket spending: impact on vulnerable beneficiaries. New York: The Commonwealth Fund, Program on Medicare's Future. Available online at www.cmwf.org/programs/medfutur/maxwell_increases_430.pdf. Accessed February 2004.

McCarthy EP, Phillips RS, Zhong Z, Drews RE, Lynn J. 2000. Dying with cancer: patients' function, symptoms, and care preferences as death approaches. *J Am Geriatr Soc.* 48:S110–121.

McCorkle R, Pasacreta JV. 2001. Enhancing caregiver outcomes in palliative care. *Cancer Control.* 8:36–45.

Medicare Payment Advisory Commission. 2003. Disease management in traditional Medicare. Statement of the Medicare Payment Advisory Commission before the Committee on Aging, U.S. Senate. November 4. Available online at www.medpac.gov/publications/congressional_testimony/110403_SenateAgingonDM.pdf. Accessed November 2003.

Medicare Prescription Drug, Improvement, and Modernization Act. 2003. Public Law 108–173. 108th Cong. December 8.

Merlis M. 2000. Caring for the frail elderly: an international review. *Health Affairs.* 19:141–149.

Metropolitan Life Insurance Company. 1999. The MetLife juggling act study: balancing caregiving with work and the cost involved. Findings from a national study by the National Alliance for Caregiving and the National Center on Women and Aging at Brandeis University. Westport, CT: MetLife Mature Market Group. Available online at www.caregiving.org/Juggling Study.pdf. Accessed February 2004.

Mezey MD, Dubler NN, Bottrell M, Mitty E, Ramsey G, Post LF, Hill T. 2001. Guidelines for end-of-life care in nursing facilities: principles and recommendations. New York: John A. Hartford Foundation Institute for Geriatric Nursing. Available online at www.hartfordign.org/resources/policy/guidelines_end_of_life.html. Accessed February 2004.

Midwest Bioethics Center. 2002. Community-state partnerships to improve end-of-life care. Available online at www.midbio.org/npo-about.htm. Accessed July 2003.

Milbank Memorial Fund and Robert Wood Johnson Foundation. 2000. Pioneer programs in palliative care: nine case studies. Available online at www.milbank.org/reports/pppc/0011pppc.html. Accessed July 2003.

Mor V, Kidder D. 1985. Cost savings in hospice: final results of the National Hospice Study. *Health Serv Res.* 20(4):407–422.

Morris JN, Mor V, Goldberg RJ, Sherwood S, Greer DS, Hiris J. 1986. The effect of treatment setting and patient characteristics on pain in terminal cancer patients: a report from the National Hospice Study. *J Chron Dis.* 39:27–35.

Moss AJ, Zareba W, Hall WJ, Klein H, Wilber DJ, Cannom DS, Daubert JP, Higgins SL, Brown MW, Andrews ML, Multicenter automatic defibrillator implantation trial II investigators. 2002. Prophylactic implantation of a defibrillator in patients with myocardial infarction and reduced ejection fraction. *N Engl J Med.* 348:877–933.

Murphy, S. 2000. Deaths: final data for 1998. National Vital Statistics Reports. 48(11). Available online at www.cdc.gov/nchs/data/nvsr/nvsr48/nvs48_11 .pdf. Accessed July 2003.

Myers S, Lynn J. 2002. The center for patient safety at the end of life: seeking reliability and safety in the care of individuals nearing the end of life with serious illness. *Topics Health Info Man.* 23(2):13–21.

National Aging Information Center. 1996. *Aging into the twenty-first century.* U.S. Administration on Aging. Washington, DC: Government Printing Office.

National Alliance for Caregiving and the American Association of Retired Persons. 1997. Family caregiving in the U.S.: findings from a national survey. Available online at www.caregiving.org/finalreport.pdf. Accessed November 2003.

National Association of State Budget Officers. 2003. Medicaid and other state healthcare issues: current trends. Available online at www.nasbo.org/ Publications/Medicaid/medicaidfeature2003.pdf. Accessed November 2003.

National Cancer Policy Board. 2001. *Improving palliative care for cancer.* Foley K, Gelband H, eds. Washington, DC: National Academies Press.

National Center for Health Statistics. 2001. Fast stats A to Z: deaths/mortality. Available online at www.cdc.gov/nchs/fastats/deaths.htm. Accessed November 2003.

———. 2002. Table 12, estimated life expectancy at birth in years, by race and sex: death-registration states, 1900–1928, and United States, 1929–2000. National Vital Statistics Reports. 51(3):33–34. December 19. Available online at www.cdc.gov/nchs/data/dvs/nvsr51_03t12.pdf. Accessed November 2003.

National Coalition for Health Care and Institute for Healthcare Improvement. 2000. Promises to keep: changing the way we provide care at the end of life. A.C.T. October. Available online at www.nchc.org/materials/studies/ EOL101200.pdf. Accessed July 2003.

———. 2002. Curing the system: stories of change in chronic illness care. A.C.T. May. Available online at www.nchc.org/materials/studies/ACT3final .pdf. Accessed July 2003.

National Council of State Boards of Nursing. 2002. National Council Licensure Examination–Registered Nurse/Practical Nurse (NCLEX-RN and NCLEX-PN) examination statistics. Statistics from years 1995–2002. Available online at www.ncsbn.org/research_stats/nclex.asp. Accessed February 2004.

National Council on Disability. 2003. National disability policy: a progress report. December 2001–December 2002. Washington, DC: National Council on Disability. Available online at www.ncd.gov/newsroom/publications/ progressreport_final.html. Accessed July 2003.

National Family Caregivers Association. 2000a. 54 million Americans involved in family caregiving last year: double the previously reported figure. Available online at www.nfcacares.org/PRSurvey2000.html. Accessed July 2003.

———. 2000b. Random sample survey of 1000 adults. Available online at www.nfcacares.org/NFC2002.stats.html. Accessed November 2003.

National Hospice and Palliative Care Organization. 2003a. 885,000 terminally ill Americans served by hospice in 2002. Press release. July. Alexandria, VA: NHPCO.

———. 2003b. NHPCO facts and figures. Available online at www.nhpco .org/files/public/Facts_Figures_Jan_03.pdf. Accessed July 2003.

National Hospice and Palliative Care Organization and Center to Advance Palliative Care. 2001. Hospital-hospice partnerships in palliative care: creating a continuum of service. Available online at www.capc.org/Filcs/ tmp_134090747.pdf. Accessed July 2003.

National Hospice Organization. 1995. An analysis of the cost savings of Medicare hospice benefit. Miami, FL: Lewin-VHI, Inc. NHO item code 712901.

National Institute for Clinical Excellence. 2003. Guidance on Cancer series. Improving supportive and palliative care for adults with cancer: manual. Consultation draft. July. Available online at www.nice.org.uk/pdf/supppalldraft manual.pdf. Accessed February 2004.

National PACE Association. 2000. PACE profile: Program of All-Inclusive Care for the Elderly. Available online at www.natlpaceassn.org/content/press/ profile_2001.asp. Accessed July 2003.

———. 2002. National PACE Association unveils new financial planning tools to aid in PACE expansion. Available online at www.natlpaceassn.org/ content/press/pr-1-23-03-.asp. Accessed November 2003.

———. 2003. What is PACE? Services. Available online at www.natlpaceassn .org/content/press/what_pace.asp. Accessed July 2003.

National Task Force on End-of-Life Care in Managed Care. 1999. Meeting the challenge: twelve recommendations for improving end-of-life care in managed care. Newton, MA: Education Development Center.

Noelker L. 2001. The backbone of the long-term-care workforce. *Generations*. 25(1):85–91.

Older Women's League (OWL). 2004. A poor prognosis: healthcare costs and aging women. Washington, DC: OWL.

Oregon Health Sciences University. 2002. The Oregon report card: improving care of the dying. Available online at www.ohsu.edu/ethics/barriers2.pdf. Accessed July 2003.

Phillips CO, Wright SM, Kern DE, Singa RM, Shepperd S, Rubin HR. 2004. Comprehensive discharge planning with postdischarge support for older patients with congestive heart failure: a meta-analysis. *JAMA.* 291:1358–1367.

Phillips DF, Sabatino CP, Long KN. 2001. Compendium of health care organization guidelines and position statements on issues related to the care of the dying. Washington DC: Last Acts. Available online at www.lastacts.org/files/publications/2001guidelinescompendium.pdf. Accessed February 2004.

Podbregar M, Voga G, Krivec B, Skale R, Gabrscek L. 2001. Should we confirm our clinical diagnostic certainty by autopsies? *Intensive Care Med.* 90: 1964–1972.

Pritchard RS, Fisher ES, Teno JM, Sharp SM, Reding DJ, Knaus WA, Wennberg JE, Lynn J. 1998. Influence of patient preferences and local health system characteristics on the place of death. SUPPORT investigators. *J Am Geriatr Soc.* 46:1242–1250.

Promoting Excellence in End-of-Life Care. 2002. Balm of Gilead Center at the Cooper Green Hospital. Available online at www.promotingexcellence.org/navigate/challenging_settings.html. Accessed July 2003.

Province MA, Hadley EC, Hornbrook MC, Lipsitz LA, Miller JP, Mulrow CD, Ory MG, Sattin RW, Tinetti ME, Wolf SL. 1995. The effects of exercise on falls in elderly patients: a preplanned meta-analysis of the FICSIT trials. *JAMA.* 273:1341–1347.

QualityHealthCare.org. 2003. Improving patient flow: the Esther project in Sweden. Available online at www.qualityhealthcare.org/QHC/Topics/Flow/PatientFlow/ImprovementStories/ImprovingPatientFlowTheEsther ProjectinSweden.htm. Accessed February 2004.

Quill TE, Byock IR. 2000. Responding to intractable terminal suffering: the role of terminal sedation and voluntary refusal of food and fluids. *Ann Intern Med.* 132:408–414.

Rabow MW, Hardie GE, Fair JM, McPhee SJ. 2000. End-of-life care content in fifty textbooks from multiple specialties. *JAMA.* 283:771–778.

Rich JS, Sox HC. 2000. Screening in the elderly: principles and practice. *Hosp Pract.* 35:45–48, 53–56.

Rich MW, Beckham V, Wittenberg C, Leven CL, Freedland KE, Carney RM. 1995. A multidisciplinary intervention to prevent the readmission of elderly patients with congestive heart failure. *N Engl J Med.* 333:1190–1195.

Rigoglioso R. 2000. Your money or your life: the financial burden of caregiving. In Levine C, ed. *Always on Call*. New York: United Hospital Fund of New York.

Rimer S. 2000. Home aides for the elderly are in short supply. *New York Times*. January 3.

Robert Wood Johnson Foundation. 2000. Overview of the chronic care model. Available online at www.improvingchroniccare.org/change/model/components.html. Accessed July 2003.

Rockwood K, Noseworth TW, Gibney RT, Konopad E, Shustack A, Stollery D, Johnston R, Grace M. 1993. One-year outcome of elderly and young patients admitted to intensive care units. *Crit Care Med*. 21:687–691.

Romer AL, Heller KS, Weissman DE, Solomon MZ, eds. 2002. *Innovations in end-of-life care: practical strategies and international perspectives*. 3 vols. Last Acts Series. New York: Liebert.

Rosalynn Carter Institute for Human Development. 2003. Advancing caregiving in America: fifteenth anniversary report. Available online at http://rci.gsw.edu/RCI_15.pdf. Accessed July 2003.

Rosenbach M, Young C. 2000. Care coordination and Medicaid managed care: emerging issues for states and managed care organizations. Policy brief. Document no. PR99–55e. Princeton, NJ: Mathematica Policy Research, Inc. Available online at www.mathematica-mpr.com/PDFs/caresum.pdf. Accessed November 2003.

Roth K, Lynn J, Zhong Z, Borum M, Dawson NV. 2000. Dying with end stage liver disease with cirrhosis: insights from SUPPORT. *J Am Geriatr Soc*. 48:122–130.

Saunders C, Clark D. 2002. *Cicely Saunders: founder of the hospice movement. Selected letters, 1959–1999*. New York: Oxford University Press.

Schulz R, Beach SR. 1999. Caregiving as a risk factor for mortality. *JAMA*. 282:2215–1419.

Scitovsky A. 1988. Medical care in the last twelve months of life: the relation between age, functional status, and medical care expenditures. *Milbank Q*. 66(4):640–660.

Selwyn PA, Forstein M. 2003. Overcoming the false dichotomy of curative vs palliative care for late-stage HIV/AIDS: "Let me live the way I want to live, until I can't." *JAMA*. 290:806–814.

Sharma R, Chan S, Liu H, Ginsberg C. 2001. *Health and health care of the Medicare population: data from the 1997 Medicare current beneficiary survey*. Rockville, MD: Westat.

Shugarman L, Campbell D, Gabel J, Bird C, Louis T, Lynn J. 2004. Differences in Medicare expenditures during the last three years of life. *JGIM*. 19:127–135.

Sieger CE, Arnold JF, Ahronheim JC. 2002. Refusing artificial nutrition and hydration: does statutory law send the wrong message? *J Am Geriatr Soc.* 50:544–550.

Singer P, Wolfson M. 2003. The best places to die: improving end of life care requires better population level data. *BMJ.* 327:173–174.

Smith TJ, Coyne P, Cassel B, Penberthy L, Hopson A, Hager MA. 2003. A high-volume specialist palliative care unit and team may reduce in-hospital end-of-life care costs. *J Palliat Med.* 6:699–705.

Smits HL, Furletti M, Vladeck BC. 2002. Palliative care: an opportunity for Medicare. New York: Institute for Medicare Practice. Available online at http://old.capc.org/content/177/177.PDF. Accessed February 2004.

Spillman B, Lubitz J. 2000. The effect of longevity on spending for acute and long-term care. *N Engl J Med.* 328:1092–1096.

State Medical Licensure Requirements and Statistics. 2003. Available online at www.ama-assn.org/ama1/pub/upload/mm/40/table14_03.pdf. Accessed July 2003.

Stevens RA. 1996. Health care in the early 1960s. *Health Care Financ Rev.* 18(2):11–22.

Stone RI. 2002. Long-term care for the elderly with disabilities: current policy, emerging trends, and implications for the twenty-first century. New York: Milbank Memorial Fund Reports.

SUPPORT Principal Investigators. 1995. A controlled trial to improve care for seriously ill hospitalized patients. Study to Understand Prognoses and Preferences for Outcomes and Risks of Treatments. *JAMA.* 274:1591–1598.

Tauber C. 1976. If nobody died of cancer . . . ? An analysis of demographic data. In *Death and dying: an examination of legislative and policy issues.* Papers from a conference cosponsored by the Health Policy Center, Georgetown University, and the American Association for the Advancement of Science. Washington, DC.

Temkin-Greener H, Mukamel DB. 2002. Predicting place of death in the Program of All-Inclusive Care for the Elderly (PACE): participant versus program characteristics. *J Am Geriatr Soc.* 50:125–135.

Tennstedt S. 1999. Family caregiving in an aging society. Report, Administration on Aging. Available online at www.aoa.gov/caregivers/FamCare.htm. Accessed July 2003.

Teno JM. 2003. Now is the time to embrace nursing homes as a place of care for dying persons. *J Palliat Med.* 6:293–296.

Teno JM, Clarridge BR, Casey V, Welch LC, Wetle T, Shield R, Mor V. 2004. Family perspectives on end-of-life care at the last place of care. *JAMA.* 291:88–93.

Teno JM, Lynn J. 1996. Putting advance-care planning into action. *J Clin Ethics.* 7:205–213.

Tolle SW, Tilden VP, Nelson CA, Dunn PM. 1998. A prospective study of the efficacy of the physician order form for life-sustaining treatment. *J Am Geriatr Soc.* 46:1097–1102.

Tuch H, Parrish P, Romer AL. 2003. Integrating palliative care into nursing homes. *J Palliat Med.* 6:297–309.

United Nations. 2002. Report of the Second World Assembly on Aging. Madrid: United Nations. April 8–12.

U.S. Bureau of Labor Statistics. 2001. *Monthly Labor Review.* Available online at www.bls.gov. Accessed November 2003.

U.S. Census Bureau. 2000. National population projections. Available online at www.census.gov/population/www/projections/natproj.html. Accessed July 2003.

U.S. Congress. 2002. Senate. Special Committee on Aging. 107th Cong. Comm. Pub. no. 107–9. Washington, DC: Government Printing Office.

U.S. Department of Health and Human Services. 1997. Office of the Inspector General. Hospice patients in nursing homes. Available online at http://oig .hhs.gov/oei/reports/oei-05-95-00250.pdf. Accessed February 2004.

———. 2000. Office of Disease Prevention and Health Promotion. Healthy people 2010: objectives for improving health. Available online at www .healthypeople.gov/document/pdf/uih/uih.pdf. Accessed February 2004.

———. 2003. Medicare enrollment: national trends, 1966–2002. Available online at cms.hhs.gov/statistics/enrollment/natltrends/hi_smi.asp. Accessed November 2003.

U.S. Department of Health and Human Services and Department of Labor. 2003. The future supply of long-term care workers in relation to the aging baby boom generation: report to Congress. Washington, DC: Government Printing Office.

U.S. General Accounting Office. 2000. Medicare: more beneficiaries use hospice

but for fewer days of care. Available online at http://frwebgate.access
.gpo.gov/cgi-bin/useftp.cgi?IPaddress=162.140.64.88&filename=he00182
.pdf&directory=/diskb/wais/data/gao. Accessed July 2003.

Veterans Affairs. 2002. Pain as the fifth vital sign: take 5. Available online at
www.va.gov/OAA/pocketcard/pain.asp. Accessed July 2003.

Veterans Health Care System. 2002. Final report for VA faculty leaders project
for improved care at the end of life. Available online at www.va.gov/
OAA/flp/Compendium/35.asp. Accessed July 2003.

Vitaliano P. 1997. Physiological and physical concomitants of caregiving. Intro-
duction to special issue. *Ann Behav Med.* 19:75–77.

Wagner EH. 1998. Chronic disease management: what will it take to improve
care for chronic illness? *Effective Clinical Practice.* 1:2–4.

Wagner EH, Davis C, Schaefer J, Von Korff M, Austin B. 1999. A survey of leading chronic disease management programs: are they consistent with the literature? *Managed Care Quarterly.* 7(3):56–66.

Walker D. 2002. Long-term care: aging baby boom generation will increase demand and burden on federal and state budgets. Statement before the Special
Committee on Aging, U.S. Senate. U.S. General Accounting Office: Government Printing Office.

Warren E, Sullivan T, Jacoby MB. 2000. Medical problems and bankruptcy fil-
ings. Social Science Electronic Publishing. Available online at http://
papers.ssrn.com/paper.taf?abstract_id=224581. Accessed July 2003.

Welch HG, Albertson PC, Nease RF, Bubolz TA, Wasson JH. 1996. Estimating
treatment benefits for the elderly: the effect of competing risks. *Ann Intern
Med.* 124:577–584.

Wenger NS, Rosenfeld K. 2001. Quality indicators for end-of-life care in vulnerable elders. *Ann Intern Med.* 135:S677–685.

Wenger NS, Shekelle PG, and the ACOVE Investigators. 2001. Assessing care
of vulnerable elders: ACOVE project overview. *Ann Intern Med.* 135:
S642–646.

Wenger NS, Solomon DH, Roth CP, MacLean CH, Saliba D, Kamberg CJ,
Rubenstein LZ, Young RT, Sloss EM, Louie R, Adams J, Chang JT, Venus
PJ, Schnelle JF, Shekelle PG. 2003. The quality of medical care provided
to vulnerable community-dwelling older patients. *Ann Intern Med.*
139:740–747.

White AJ, Abel Y, Kidder D. 2000. Evaluation of the Program of All-Inclusive
Care for the Elderly demonstration: a comparison of the PACE capitation
rates to projected costs in the first year of enrollment. Final report. Available

online at www.cms.hhs.gov/researchers/reports/2000/white.pdf. Accessed November 2003.

Wilkinson AM. 1996. Past research on long-term care case management demonstrations. In Newcomer RJ, Wilkinson AM, eds., *Annual review of gerontology and geriatrics*, vol. 16, *Focus on managed care and quality assurance: integrating acute and chronic care*, 104–111. New York: Springer Publishing.

Wilner, MA. 2000. Toward a stable and experienced caregiver workforce. *Generations*. 24:60–65.

Wolff J, Starfield B, Anderson G. 2002. Prevalence, expenditures, and complications of multiple chronic conditions in the elderly. *Arch Intern Med.* 162:2269–2276.

World Health Organization (WHO). 1990. Cancer pain relief and palliative care. Report of World Health Organization Expert Committee. Technical Series no. 804.

———. 2004. *Better palliative care for older people*. Davies E, Higginson IJ, eds. Geneva: World Health Organization Europe.

Zhong Z, Lynn J. 1999. The Lamont/Christakis article reviewed. *Oncology*. 13:1172–1173.

Zuckerman C, Mackinnon A. 1998. The challenge of caring for patients near the end of life: findings from the hospital palliative care initiative. New York: United Hospital Fund.

Index

Page numbers in *italics* indicate figures and tables.

Compositor:	Binghamton Valley Composition, LLC
Indexer:	Victoria Baker
Illustrator:	Bill Nelson
Text:	10/15 Janson
Display:	Janson
Printer and binder:	Maple-Vail Manufacturing Group